Developing Person-Centred Cultures in Healthcare Education and Practice

Developing Person-Centred Cultures in Healthcare Education and Practice

An Essential Guide

Edited by

BRENDAN McCORMACK

Susan Wakil Professor of Nursing, Head of School and Dean
The Susan Wakil School of Nursing and Midwifery
(inc. Sydney Nursing School)
Faculty of Medicine and Health
The University of Sydney, Australia

WILEY Blackwell

The right of Brendan McCormack to be identified as the editorial material in this work has been asserted in accordance with law.

Registered Offices
John Wiley & Sons, Inc., 111 River Street, Hoboken, NJ 07030, USA
John Wiley & Sons Ltd, The Atrium, Southern Gate, Chichester, West Sussex, PO19 8SQ, UK

For details of our global editorial offices, customer services, and more information about Wiley products visit us at www.wiley.com.

Wiley also publishes its books in a variety of electronic formats and by print-on-demand. Some content that appears in standard print versions of this book may not be available in other formats.

Library of Congress Cataloging-in-Publication Data Applied for:
Paperback ISBN: 9781119913863
ePDF: 9781119913870
ePUB: 9781119913887

Cover Design: Wiley
Cover Image: © freshidea/Adobe Stock Photos

Set in 10/12pt STIXTwoText by Straive, Pondicherry, India
Printed and bound by CPI Group (UK) Ltd, Croydon, CR0 4YY

C9781119913863_080324

Dedication

We dedicate this book to the life and works of Professor Jan Dewing (1961–2022). Jan was a member of the original project team, and while she began the journey with us, she was unable to see it through to the end. Jan's commitment to and passion for person-centred learning have been woven through the project to develop the first pan-European curriculum framework for the education of person-centred healthcare professionals. Her legacy lives on in this and other works and her voice permeates the rich tapestry of person-centredness we are committed to as authors.

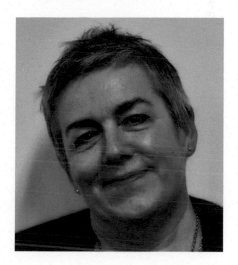

Some of us are ... in the paradoxical position of enjoying or even taking for granted significant privilege while also being committed to addressing it in some way or other. This leaves us ... asking: *How can I/we deploy the benefits we have amassed to meaningfully contribute against the oppression of others?* (Dewing 2020)

Contents

List of Contributors

Donna Brown
Senior Lecturer in Nursing
School of Nursing and Paramedic Science
Ulster University
Belfast, Northern Ireland

Gobnait Byrne
Assistant Professor
School of Nursing and Midwifery
Trinity College Dublin
Dublin, Ireland

Shaun Cardiff
Senior Lecturer
Fontys University of Applied Sciences
Eindhoven, The Netherlands

Neil Cook
Professor of Nursing
Head of School of Nursing and Paramedic Science
Ulster University
Belfast, Northern Ireland

Caroline Dickson
Senior Lecturer in Nursing
School of Health Sciences
Queen Margaret University
Edinburgh, Scotland

Stephanie Dunleavy
Senior Lecturer in Nursing
School of Nursing and Paramedic Science
Ulster University
Belfast, Northern Ireland

Helle Kristine Falkenberg
Professor
Department of Optometry, Radiography and Lighting Design
Faculty of Health and Social Sciences
University of South-Eastern Norway
Notodden, Norway

Erna Haraldsdottir
Professor
Deputy Head, Division of Nursing and Paramedic Science
Director, Centre for Person-centred Practice Research
School of Health Sciences
Queen Margaret University
Edinburgh, Scotland

Sergej Kmetec
Teaching Assistant
Faculty of Health Sciences
University of Maribor
Maribor, Slovenia

Mateja Lorber
Associate Professor and Dean of Faculty
Faculty of Health Sciences
University of Maribor
Maribor, Slovenia

Ruth Magowan
Interim Head of Division of Nursing and Paramedic Science
Senior Lecturer
School of Health Sciences
Queen Margaret University
Edinburgh, Scotland

Tanya McCance
Mona Grey Professor of Nursing
Research and Development
School of Nursing and Para-
medic Science
Ulster University
Belfast, Northern Ireland

Brendan McCormack
The Susan Wakil Professor of Nursing;
Head of School and Dean, Susan Wakil
School of Nursing and Midwifery
(Sydney Nursing School) Faculty of
Medicine and Health, The University
of Sydney, Australia; Professor II,
Østfold University College, Norway;
Extraordinary Professor, University
of Pretoria, South Africa; Professor of
Nursing, Maribor University, Slovenia;
Visiting Professor, Ulster University;
Adjunct Professor, Zealand University
Hospital/University of Southern
Denmark

Deidre O'Donnell
Senior Lecturer
School of Nursing and Paramedic
Science
Ulster University
Belfast, Northern Ireland

Amanda Phelan
Professor in Ageing and Community
Nursing
School of Nursing and Midwifery
Trinity College Dublin
Dublin, Ireland

Gregor Štiglic
Professor
Faculty of Health Sciences
University of Maribor
Maribor, Slovenia

Siri Tønnessen
Head of Research and Professor
Lovisenberg Diaconal University
College
Oslo, Norway
Professor II, Department of Nursing
and Health Sciences, Faculty of Health
and Social Sciences, University of
South-Eastern Norway
Notodden, Norway

Famke van Lieshout
Associate Professor
Knowledge Centre Value-oriented
Professionalisation
University of Applied Sciences
Utrecht, The Netherlands

Foreword

There is consensus that healthcare systems need to be more person centred. People accessing healthcare services, caregivers and carers have all called for a shift towards person-centred principles based on mutual respect and collaboration between them and health professionals.

Despite stakeholders and policy documents supporting the implementation of person-centred healthcare, the process is slow and unclear in many countries. Thus, students in nursing, medicine and health programmes must be better prepared with theoretical and practical knowledge to practise and further develop this philosophy after completing their education. Unfortunately, university curricula in healthcare and medicine often lack philosophical, pedagogical and practical content about person-centredness. Dedicated course leaders and teachers wanting to share their knowledge of person-centred healthcare with students often find a lack of governance and support at university and department levels. It is far too uncommon to find institutional boards and student representatives in higher education institutions who have decided that the ethos and practice of person-centred healthcare must be integrated into the entire educational process. This attitude might be because there is no systematic and rigorous methodology for educating students and concerned clinicians in this field.

Therefore, the Universal Curriculum Framework for Person-centred Healthcare Practitioner Education presented in this book is an applauded endeavour to equip students to practise person-centredness in care, particularly in changing healthcare systems. The curriculum framework was developed by researchers and specialists in healthcare and education representing several European countries with diverse health systems. The project sought to advance the development of person-centred healthcare through an interdisciplinary curriculum to educate future healthcare practitioners and their supervisors, mentors and facilitators. Because person-centred principles and shared values frame the curriculum, the generic design of the curriculum also makes it useful outside Europe.

The authors identify a set of thematic actions to help shape how shared values influence the effective functioning of a team and contribute to cultivating a healthy learning culture. Respecting self-determination and negotiated autonomy are central to a person-centred ethos, focusing on working *with* rather than *on* persons. The values that are fundamental to the work of the educational setting, whether academic or clinical, are operationalised through the curriculum framework. The curriculum framework is particularly useful as it conveys the ethical and philosophical content of person-centred healthcare and provides an implementation strategy for the curriculum with practical actions, methods and tools.

I highly recommend this book because the Universal Curriculum Framework for Person-centred Healthcare Practitioner Education focuses on a person-centred philosophy and practice and extends beyond a vague understanding of this approach, helping all educators to develop the knowledge and skills in learners of person-centredness in healthcare.

Inger Ekman RN, PhD
Senior Professor, University of Gothenburg, Sweden
November 2023

Acknowledgements

The writing team of this book is grateful for the following support that has made this project possible.

The European Commission Erasmus + Program Call 2019 Round 1 KA2 – Cooperation for innovation and the exchange of good practices; KA203 – Strategic Partnerships for higher education FormId KA203-990E7AB4. AGREEMENT NUMBER- 2019-1-UK01-KA203 061970 for supporting the development project (the First Pan-European Curriculum Framework for Educating Health Care Practitioners in Person-centred Healthcare) that has informed the content of this book. However, the authors of this book confirm that the views and practices presented in this book are those of the authors and do not represent the views or practices of the funding agency.

All the participants in the development project that has informed the content of this book. Participants in the project came from all over the world and participated in a variety of engagement events that resulted in the development of the first Pan-European Curriculum Framework for Educating Healthcare Practitioners in Person-centred Healthcare. That framework shapes the structure and focus of this book. We are truly grateful for the time and energy they gave to this work and in helping to shape the future of person-centred healthcare.

Professor Angie Titchen and Professor Jan Dewing, who along with Professor Brendan McCormack wrote the first edition of *Practice Development Workbook for Nursing, Health and Social Care Teams* (Wiley Blackwell Publishers, 2014) and from which some of the activities included in this book have been derived. Jan started out on this journey with us, but sadly her untimely death meant she was unable to complete it.

All the colleagues, friends and family who supported us through this project. We undertook most of the work associated with the development project (the first Pan-European Curriculum Framework for Educating Health Care Practitioners in Person-centred Healthcare) throughout the Covid period. This required considerable pivoting by the project team to ensure the work could continue. We were supported in those endeavours by a variety of colleagues, friends and family members who helped us along the way. Thank you.

CHAPTER 1

Introduction

INTRODUCTION

In this introductory chapter, we provide an overview of the collaborative work we have engaged in to create the first person-centred curriculum framework to inform the development of curricula to educate healthcare practitioners. We provide an overview of the need for such a framework as well as sharing the systematic and rigorous methodology we adopted in our work. We demonstrate the iterative and reflexive approach we adopted to the development of the curriculum framework. Finally, we present the full Universal Curriculum Framework for Person-centred Healthcare Practitioner Education.

The major content of this chapter is drawn from previously published papers written by all the co-authors of this chapter. We have summarised and adapted the text from these previously published papers to present a synthesis of that work and introduce the reader to the curriculum framework itself. The complete collection of papers underpinning this chapter is listed in Table 1.1 and we would encourage you to visit this collection of papers for a deep understanding of the research and each stage of the development process that led to the finalised curriculum framework.

PERSON-CENTRED HEALTHCARE POLICY AND PRACTICE

Person-centredness, underpinned by robust philosophical and theoretical concepts, has an increasingly solid footprint in policy and practice, but research and education lag behind. In the first phase of the curriculum framework development project, we considered the emergence of person-centredness, including person-centred care and how it is positioned in healthcare policy around the world, while recognising our dominant philosophical positioning in Western philosophy, concepts and theories (Phelan et al. 2020). We critically reviewed the published literature for the period 2016 and

TABLE 1.1   Published Papers on Which this Chapter is Based.

Cook, N.F., Brown, D., O'Donnell, D. et al. (2022) The Person-centred Curriculum Framework: a universal curriculum framework for person-centred healthcare practitioner education. International Practice Development Journal 12 (Special Issue), Article 4. https://doi.org/10.19043/12Suppl.004

Dickson, C., van Lieshout, F., Kmetec, S. et al. (2020) Developing philosophical and pedagogical principles for a pan-European person-centred curriculum framework. International Practice Development Journal 10(2) (Special Issue). http://dx.doi.org/10.19043/ipdj.10Suppl2.004

McCormack, B. (2020) Educating for a person-centred future – the need for curriculum innovation. International Practice Development Journal 10 (Special Issue). http://dx.doi.org/10.19043/ipdj.10Suppl2.001

McCormack, B. (2022) Educating for a person-centred future – the need for curriculum innovation. International Practice Development Journal 12 (Special Issue). www.fons.org/library/journal/volume12-suppl/editorial

McCormack, B., Magowan, R., O'Donnell, D. et al. (2022) Developing a Person-centred Curriculum Framework: a whole-systems methodology. International Practice Development Journal 12 (Special Issue), Article 2. https://doi.org/10.19043/ipdj.12suppl.002

O'Donnell, D., McCormack, B., McCance, T. and McIlfatrick, S. (2020) A meta-synthesis of person-centredness in nursing curricula. International Practice Development Journal 10(2) (Special Issue). http://dx.doi.org/10.19043/ipdj.10Suppl2.002

O'Donnell, D., Dickson, C.A.W., Phelan, A. et al. (2022) A mixed methods approach to the development of a Person-centred Curriculum Framework: surfacing person-centred principles and practices. International Practice Development Journal 12 (Special Issue), Article 3. https://doi.org/10.19043/ipdj.12Suppl.003

Phelan, A., McCormack, B., Dewing, J. et al. (2020) Review of developments in person-centred healthcare. International Practice Development Journal 10(3) (Special Issue). http://dx.doi.org/10.19043/ipdj.10Suppl2.003

2021 to show how person-centred healthcare has evolved over this time. We drew on published evidence of person-centred healthcare developments, as well as information gathered from key stakeholders who engaged with us in this project as partner organisations. We identified five themes underpinning the literature and stakeholder perspectives.

1. Policy development for transformation.
2. Participatory strategies for public engagement.
3. Healthcare integration and co-ordination strategies.
4. Frameworks for practice.
5. Process and outcome measurement.

These themes reflect the World Health Organization's global perspective on people-centred and integrated healthcare and give some indication of development priorities as we continue to develop person-centred healthcare systems. However, our review methods also revealed the need for intentional development of individuals and teams as person-centred practitioners within pre- and postregistration programmes. The centrality of caring relationships and possessing holistic care skills is highlighted, but the day-to-day challenges experienced in practice result in the context in which learning takes place not being supportive of the developments needed. Therefore, if the global developments highlighted are to be sustained and developed at scale, then we need many role models of person-centred practice integrated at every level of the healthcare system who can facilitate person-centred learning cultures, wherever such learning takes place.

The need for healthcare education programmes to plan strategically for a workforce that is ready to respond appropriately is obvious, and education curricula need to be innovative and proactive in this respect. In practice, this 'reality' may seem unreal, as evidence from service user feedback, patient experience surveys and patient/family outcome data continues to suggest that only 'modest' improvements in patient experience have been achieved, despite more than 20 years of service improvement, quality improvement and practice developments. While there has been major investment into such improvements, as well as into patient safety (and yes, patients are safer – in hospitals at least), these data have not significantly changed over the years.

Despite these best efforts, there is little evidence of fundamental change in the core cultural characteristics of healthcare practice, and some commentators argue (drawing on culture theory as an explanatory device) that most person-centred developments focus on the artefacts of practice rather than on the core values that drive health and social care delivery. O'Donnell et al. (2020) highlighted the lack of a consistent focus on person-centred principles, even in curricula that purport to have person-centredness as their underpinning framework. At best, person-centredness is used as a heuristic for containing a diverse range of principles, processes and practices in teaching and learning, rather than being an explicit conceptual or theoretical framework informing all stages of education delivery. Although there are few examples of professional education curricula for healthcare practitioners that adequately prepare them to work in a person-centred way, they are expected to graduate from their professional programmes with the qualities and attributes of a person-centred practitioner.

It is the drive to address these ongoing challenges in developing person-centred healthcare services that motivated us to undertake the research that is the bedrock of this book. The work began in 2019 when McCormack and Dewing published a position statement on person-centredness in the curriculum. This position statement formed the basis of the case of need and the detailed funding proposal submitted to the European Commission Erasmus + Strategic Partnerships for Higher Education funding stream (KA203-990E7AB4). The research and development work undertaken is all in the public domain (Table 1.1). However, being cognisant of our earlier commentary on the challenges associated with making person-centredness real in the curriculum, we were committed not just to providing a curriculum framework but also to helping make sense of the framework through practical actions, methods and tools. So, this book provides practical applications and, if worked with, an implementation strategy for the curriculum framework developed by the project team who are also the co-authors of this book.

DEVELOPMENT OF A UNIVERSAL CURRICULUM FRAMEWORK FOR PERSON-CENTRED HEALTHCARE PRACTITIONER EDUCATION

The findings from the evidence synthesised by Phelan et al. (2020) and O'Donnell et al. (2020) and the previous work undertaken by the International Community of Practice for Person-centred Practice (PcP-ICoP)[1] in developing a position statement for person-centredness in nursing and healthcare curricula (McCormack and Dewing 2019) were the impetus for developing a person-centred curriculum framework for educating healthcare professionals, supported by funding from the European Union Erasmus + Strategic Partnerships for Higher Education Programme (Project ID KA203-990E7AB4). The project partners were Trinity College Dublin, Ireland; Fontys University of Applied Sciences, The Netherlands; Ulster University, Northern Ireland; University of Maribor, Slovenia; University of South-Eastern Norway; and Queen Margaret University Edinburgh, Scotland. The overall aim of this project was to advance the development of person-centred healthcare through an interdisciplinary curriculum to educate future healthcare practitioners and their supervisors, mentors and facilitators.

We worked in a systematic way as partner organisations, using best practices in project management, stakeholder engagement and process monitoring. Ensuring that continuous and detailed stakeholder analysis addressed the needs of different stakeholders, these were mapped against key areas of activity as the project progressed. This systematic approach was enhanced by our shared values, agreed ways of working and clarity of roles and responsibilities, as well as a timeline for key deliverables. The use of a logic model of decision making also ensured that all activities were linked to project objectives, outcomes and outputs and to quality assessment, impact and dissemination strategies. We drew upon our collective continuing networks to enable the active engagement of a broad range of interested parties with the project activities. A project advisory board oversaw the work of the project and was drawn from experts by experience, leaders in the field of person-centred healthcare, curriculum developers, higher education funding bodies, healthcare policy agencies, evaluation researchers and healthcare professional representative bodies.

In addition to the review of global developments in person-centred healthcare (Phelan et al. 2020) to contextually position the project, we undertook three

---

[1] The International Community of Practice for Person-centred Practice – Community Interest Company(PcP-ICoP CIC) is an international community of academics and healthcare providers who are interested in advancing knowledge in the field of person-centred practice. Note here that 'practice' is taken as being in any field: care, education, research, management, policy, etc. The ICoP co-ordinates a programme of research and scholarship, and supports collaborative publications and presentations as well as a thriving community of practice for doctoral candidates and postdoctoral academics who are all committed to researching and developing aspects of person-centredness. All the members are engaged in teaching and learning, research, scholarship and quality improvement activities connected to person-centred healthcare. Visit www.pcp-icop.org for further information.

further phases of work towards developing a person-centred curriculum framework for educating healthcare professionals.

- Developing philosophical and pedagogical curriculum framework principles.
- Designing a curriculum framework development methodology.
- Designing a person-centred curriculum framework for educating healthcare professionals.

Developing Philosophical and Pedagogical Curriculum Framework Principles

A participative hermeneutic praxis methodology was created as a means of systematically guiding the co-creation of the principles underpinning the curriculum framework development. The process, consistent with person-centredness, was grounded in respect for personhood and mutuality. Phases and steps in the process were realised progressively, guided by a form of practical reasoning and moral intent. Each partner participated actively in the process that was characterised by critical and creative dialogues. Understanding and respect for each cultural background and language used were key to the process, as well as mutual adequacy and growth for individuals and the team. Through mutual processes of inquiring about *what* is significant in the context of the project and *how* to apply it in a situation, a co-constructed praxis design was generated.

Further methodological guidance was sought from the philosophical tradition of hermeneutics. Using the hermeneutics perspective of Gadamer and Dutt (1993), we aimed to develop an understanding of the study focus using the subjective interpretation of individuals as well as the collective consciousness of the group. Understanding arises from repetitive reading of the various datasets; being open to the concepts being sought; being aware of our prejudices and critiquing/allowing them to be critiqued in light of newly formulated meanings (Boomer and McCormack 2010).

Two processes key to understanding the data were the hermeneutic circle (Heidegger 1967) and the fusion of horizons (Gadamer and Dutt 1993). The hermeneutic circle is the idea that understanding of the data as a whole is established by reference to the individual parts and understanding the parts by reference to the whole. Neither the whole dataset nor the parts can be understood without reference to the other, and hence a circle of constant movement between the parts and the whole is established. Interpretation is never free of presupposition; what we know cognitively, precognitively and feel (preunderstanding) is the frame of reference ('horizon') from which a person starts. During dialogue with others, everyone starts from their own horizon and through listening, questioning and theorising, these personal or cultural 'horizons' were challenged, became broader and fused with others, resulting in a new, more encompassing understanding of what is needed to prepare practitioners for person-centred practice.

Approach Used to Collaboratively Design Curriculum Framework Principles

The overall process consisted of three co-designed phases that demonstrated movement between the parts and the whole, intersecting on several occasions of critical dialogue.

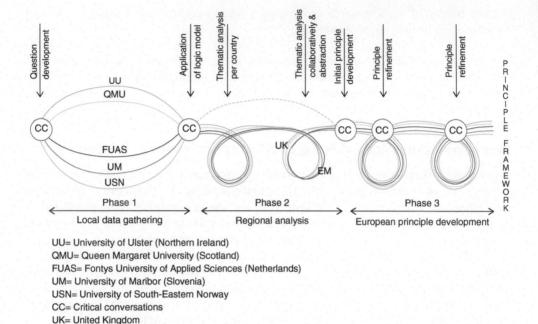

FIGURE 1.1   Overview of participative hermeneutic praxis methodology.

Critical conversations aimed at collaboratively reflecting on and working with the data and creating the opportunity to fuse horizons were key processes (Figure 1.1).

- *Phase 1 – 'Moving from the whole ...'*: the project group co-constructed questions to engage with stakeholders in the UK, Netherlands, Norway and Slovenia to collect perspectives on what is needed to enable person-centred practice to become a reality. Each project partner used differing methods to engage with stakeholders to capture their views.
- *Phase 2 – '... to the parts ...'*: moving through the hermeneutic circle, the intention of the second phase was to understand and create new meaning, through fusion of horizons. Multiple rounds of data analysis were conducted. A first step was a thematic analysis in each country, then a collective analysis of the whole dataset with partners. The third step was an abstract level of data analysis in which the partners engaged in theorising, using the Person-centred Practice Framework and Hart's (2019) purpose, life and system world model. Methods used were creative workshops with all six partners and working in subgroups to synthesise data, identify and map themes within the datasets through moving up and down different levels of abstraction.
- *Phase 3 – '...and back to the whole...'*: during this phase, the analysed data were used for development of the principles framework which would inform the development of a person-centred curriculum framework in the next phase of the project.

'A person-centred curriculum is person centred if it is transformative (purpose), grounded in a philosophy of pragmatism (systems world) and enables all learners to co-construct (lifeworld) and experience connectivity with oneself, other persons and contexts (lifeworld) throughout their personal learning journey'

FIGURE 1.2   Core principles underpinning a person-centred curriculum.

The hermeneutic process continued with multiple rounds of identification and refinement of principles. A small workgroup with representatives from the different countries/partners led this process. Multiple draft versions of the framework were shared with partners for critique. As part of this process, the principles were checked with original stakeholder data to ensure consistency.

Through these iterative processes, consensus was reached about the core principles underpinning a person-centred curriculum (Figure 1.2). To be person-centred in healthcare, attention needs to be paid to a triadic relationship between the practitioner's competencies and commitment, together with the local environment. There also needs to be a whole-system understanding and support for person-centredness. Practitioners who 'care with' others, rather than 'care for' or just 'about' others, are essential. They need to acknowledge and work with the whole person and to be reflective and a good communicator. There needs to be reciprocal understanding and practitioners need to be able to reveal discrepancies between actual and espoused practices through critical reflection. Practitioners need to feel a responsibility for being competent and courageous in challenging and changing their practice and so championing person-centred practice. There is also commitment to living person-centredness and to connect with (those upholding) related perspectives. This requires facilitators of learning and learners to role model person-centred ways of being and to live out person-centred ideals in their interactions and in navigating conflicting values, structures and policies. Both the theory and practice of person-centredness need to be understood in order for a person to become a proficient person-centred practitioner.

There needs to be a local person-centred environment and culture valuing staff diversity and expertise, sensitive to and understanding experiences, feelings and needs of all stakeholders. A collaborative inclusive and participative approach in the development of any relationship and student-teacher nexus is needed. However, issues of culture, context and the behaviours of people, across healthcare and academic settings, act as barriers to individual learning. Generally, a whole-system approach is needed in organisational thinking and design, in which there is minimal bureaucracy and structures and processes act as servants to the lifeworld and relationships of persons and not the other way round, which is often more common. A supportive meso-/macro-context that provides guidance for developments in effective learning environments is essential, for example for critical conversations with organisational leaders and managers and with experienced clinical and academic staff where boundaries are removed. In this context, the focus could be on coping with challenges to person-centred practice, as well as reflecting on the intended outcomes of innovations in person-centred practice, ultimately enhancing student (and practitioner) opportunities to learn and practise in more person-centred ways in a safe environment. Learning can only happen in an environment where the evidence and knowledge of clinical and academic staff are contemporaneous. This set of philosophical dimensions, methodological and pedagogical principles for person-centred curriculum design is shown in Table 1.2.

Designing a Curriculum Framework Development Methodology

We adapted the 7S methodology of Waterman et al. (1980) to design the person-centred curriculum framework. Originally developed as an organisational analysis framework, the 7S methodology deals with snapshots of complex systems, usually as a means of change management. These complex systems are contemporary, or desired. Using the 7S methodology assists with the identification and alignment of the seven elements to achieve a desired future state; this can be, for example, through the addition, supplementation or enhancement of some or all of the seven elements. Therefore, although Waterman et al. describe the methodology as a 'gap analysis', it is perhaps better to see it as a *thematic analysis* permitting identification of areas of deficit that can be augmented/amended to align all elements of the system, but which can also identify areas of 'added value' which can be realigned or employed elsewhere. 7S can also potentially assist with the relationships (functional or dysfunctional) between the elements, meaning it is more powerful than a 'simple' gap analysis, i.e. where there are two fixed points that need to be brought closer together. Gap analysis often focuses on 'bad practice' or 'what is wrong' that causes the gap to exist, but use of the 7S methodology allows identification of 'good practice across the whole system' through the thematic analysis approach.

The 7S methodology recognises seven elements of a system and divides these into 'hard' and 'soft' elements (Figure 1.3).

The 'hard' elements are:

1. strategy
2. structure
3. systems.

The 'soft' elements are:

4. shared values
5. skills
6. style
7. staff.

Shared values are core to all the elements and Figure 1.3 shows the interconnectedness and interdependence of the elements and the centrality of shared values. It also highlights that a change in one element can affect all the others. All elements of the 7S methodology are equally important to the functioning of the complex system, and they are all mutually related and interdependent: they form and operate as a web.

TABLE 1.2 Principles for Person-centred Curriculum Design.

Framework purpose, lifeworld, systems world	**Methodological principle**: the philosophical approach to curriculum design	**Pedagogical principles**: teaching, learning and assessment (TLA) and the context of learning
Purpose (person-centred outcomes)	**Philosophical dimension**: transformative	A person-centred approach to teaching, learning and assessment
	Methodological principle: curriculum is transformative and enables journeying through knowing, doing, being and becoming a competent and committed person-centred practitioner	**TLA strategies:**

TLA strategies:

1. Learning is holistic, focusing on multiple ways of knowing the whole person

2. Teaching, learning and assessment approaches guide learners journeying through knowing, doing, being and becoming a person-centred practitioner

3. Learning is progressive: progressing to the point where person-centredness is embodied as a learner, practitioner and leader of person-centred practice

4. Reflexivity is integral to active learning approaches, enabling movement from preconsciousness, through consciousness to critical consciousness, creating perspective transformation as a person-centred practitioner

5. Active learning enables new insights to become translated into actions to be tested and evaluated in practice

6. Eclectic teaching, learning and assessment strategies draw on critical creativity as well as technical-rational approaches to enable learning to be systematic and incremental with deliberate intent

7. Learners and facilitators learn together with and from each other, shaping new knowledge

Learning environment:

8. Person-centredness is embodied by all involved in and supportive of the curriculum

9. Learners experience and practise person-centredness

10. Learners are helped to become brave in challenging practice

(Continued)

TABLE 1.2 (Continued)

Lifeworld 1 (health-care relationships)	**Philosophical dimension:** co-constructed	**TLA strategies:**

Philosophical dimension:
co-constructed

Methodological principle:
a co-constructionist approach to curriculum design and implementation where the curriculum is flexible and adaptive to the learner

TLA strategies:

1. Learning is participative, inclusive and collaborative in all learning relationships
2. Opportunities for creating shared social responsibility, in co-creation of curricula, based on moral intents
3. TLA are sensitive and responsive to these mutual learning needs which are open to negotiation
4. Learners determine their own learning pathway
5. Learners at different stages of the learning journey are encouraged to learn together
6. Learners and teaching staff actively engage in mutual learning

Learning environment:

1. A culture of safety, relationships and learning is co-created
2. Safe learning environments are created for exploration, shared understanding, decision making and action
3. Preconditions are created by those with a stake in the curriculum to co-create the processes necessary for curricular design
4. Educators show courage, humility and vulnerability in the facilitation of learning
5. Practice-based mentors are engaged as part of the programme team
6. Freedom of individual expression is encouraged
7. Taking risks and (calculated or intentional/moral) experimentation are encouraged, supported and subject to wider critique through reflective processes
8. Practitioner and service user experiences are evaluation criteria used to critique and promote knowing, doing, being and becoming a person-centred practitioner
9. Safe spaces evolve into brave spaces in which everyone feels comfortable with diversity and experiences respect, inclusion and emotional support

| Lifeworld 2 (learner relationships) | **Philosophical dimension:** relational

Methodological principle: curriculum encourages connectivity with oneself, other persons and contexts | **TLA strategies:**
1. Fundamentals of person-centredness are continually revisited
2. Learning involves maximising generation and transmission of multiple sources of evidence to support knowledge of person-centred practice
3. Person-centred facilitation is embedded in TLA approaches
4. Social learning and meaning making are encouraged through safe communicative spaces
5. Opportunities are given to reflect on relationships with others and with materials and space

Learning environment:
6. Person-centredness is embodied by everyone engaging and communicating authentically
7. Critical questioning is embedded in learning processes
8. Caring relationships that foster mutuality are created
9. Diversity is welcomed and respected
10. All involved in the curriculum accept moral responsibility for others |
| Systems world (environmental/organisational structures, processes, administration) to create a systems world that supports the life-world in realising purpose | **Philosophical dimension:** pragmatic

Methodological principle: curriculum is built on a philosophy of pragmatism | **TLA strategies:**
1. Theory and practice are intertwined
2. Debate and discussion create opportunities to deconstruct idealism vs realism
3. Engaging in enquiry-based learning to become facilitators within the whole and multi-layered contexts
4. Learning is embedded in movement between local, national and global contexts
5. Generation and sharing of multiple sources of evidence will support the development of competence (knowledge, skills and attitudes) in a person-centred way |

(Continued)

TABLE 1.2 (Continued)

6. Learners consider themselves to be agents of social change
7. Embracing, working and being comfortable with complexity through enquiry-based learning
8. Ongoing evaluation of learning in relation to ever changing practice milieu

Learning environment:

1. Communicative spaces create opportunities for social learning and meaning making
2. Safe spaces evolve into brave spaces
3. Learners understand the relevance of person-centred practice through contextualised learning within real-life experiences

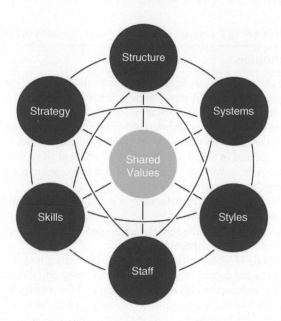

FIGURE 1.3 7S Methodology (www.mindtools.com/pages/article/newSTR_91.htm).

While the methodology was designed from an organisational science perspective, we adapted it to a healthcare context, i.e. a thematic analysis of existing healthcare curricula. Thus, it was vital that we were clear about definitions and translation of the elements from organisational science to healthcare, and between languages and healthcare settings. We needed to be precise in understanding terms and employed contextual translation techniques wherever necessary. Our adaptation process is set out in McCormack et al. (2022) and our adapted definitions of the seven elements are shown in Table 1.3 and Figure 1.4.

All elements of the 7S methodology are equally important to the functioning of the whole complex system, and they are all mutually related and interdependent, i.e. a web. Using this approach enables a thorough systematic analysis of key 'core' themes to be derived. Using the 7S methodology facilitated an analysis of the current situation (the extent to which existing curricula are person-centred) and the desired future situation (person-centred curriculum framework). We earlier presented a set of principles (philosophical, theoretical and methodological) that set out our 'desired future' person-centred healthcare curriculum framework based on the work of Dickson et al. (2020). In establishing a methodology for developing a curriculum framework, we needed to determine the extent to which existing curricula already matched these principles or were unique and thus offered a new perspective.

Being clear about the purpose of the desired curriculum framework and agreement about the shared values that would influence the other six components of the 7S methodology were critical factors in designing the detail of the methodology.

1. *Purpose.* What is the purpose of our desired complex system (the ideal, person-centred healthcare curriculum), and of the whole curriculum framework? At the

TABLE 1.3 The McKinsey 7S Framework with Adapted Definitions of Each Element.

Element	Definition
Strategy	This is the whole curriculum framework that identifies the unique selling point (USP) of the programme and what makes it unique, and thus attractive to potential students
Structure	How the curriculum is structured (modules/units/courses) to achieve the curriculum intentions as well as how the school/faculty/department is organised in terms of its structures to deliver the curriculum, including student/stakeholder engagement and processes to meet the intended regulatory requirements and quality standards
Systems	Teaching, learning and assessment methods used to achieve the stated curriculum outcomes
Shared values	The core values of the school/faculty/department and how these are made explicit in the curriculum
Style	The style of leadership used to deliver the curriculum
Staff	The general capabilities of the team with responsibility for delivering the curriculum, the skill mix of the team and the support for staff development to deliver the curriculum, i.e. the make-up of the team, its 'fit' with the curriculum intentions and staff support to deliver curriculum outcomes
Skills	The actual knowledge, expertise, skills and competence of the academic team with responsibility for delivering the curriculum

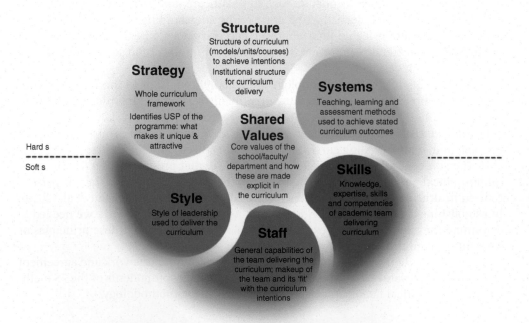

FIGURE 1.4 The adapted 7S methodological framework.

heart of this question is the need for an agreed definition of 'curriculum framework'. Such an agreed definition acts as an 'anchor' for the analysis of curricula and ensures we are analysing curricula with the same focus in mind. We developed a definition of person-centred curriculum, focusing on the idea of a 'shared curriculum' (Figure 1.5). This definition is wide enough to allow for the whole-system analysis envisaged and makes clear that this is an enterprise involving more actors than just students/teachers, because multiple actors have an investment/stake in the system. The 7S methodology therefore provides an analytical methodology permitting analysis of existing shared curriculum frameworks to identify elements that do/do not conform to our desired common goal of supporting the design, delivery and evaluation of person-centred healthcare education. In accepting this definition, we then extrapolated the underpinning shared values of the curriculum framework.

2. *Shared values* (Figure 1.6). In this project, we determined that it was not up to us to identify the values we wanted to see evidenced or to prescribe a set of values that we then go looking for. Instead, what we wanted to identify were the values that are central to the work of the department/school/faculty and how these are operationalised through the curriculum framework. The values should be consistent with how we define a person-centred culture aligned with the Person-centred Practice Framework (McCormack and McCance 2017) which informs the overall Erasmus project.

> A Shared Curriculum Framework (SCF) is a complex system comprising facilitators of shared learning in community, whose actions contribute to a common goal of supporting the design, delivery and evaluation of person-centred healthcare education [globally]. The use of a SCF creates consistency across education programmes, generates foundations for research and development, and supports the creation of pedagogical tools (teaching, learning, and evaluation) that align with the underpinning principles of the framework.

FIGURE 1.5   Curriculum framework definition.

> 'A person-centred culture enables effective engagement based on the formation and fostering of healthful relationships between all persons. It has explicit values of respect for persons' self-determination, mutual respect and understanding. It creates the conditions for all persons to engage in continuous development and self/group/community/societal transformation' (McCormack et al., 2021: 19).

FIGURE 1.6   Person-centred culture defined.
Source: Adapted from McCormack et al., 2021, p. 19.

3. *How this worked in practice*. The purpose and values act as the 'anchor' for operationalising the methodology. Common in management science is the use of a 'checklist' of questions to complete the 7S system analysis. We developed a list of questions to guide our analysis processes (see Table 1.4).

The questions shown in Table 1.4 were used to build a database to undertake curriculum analysis and guide the next stage of the project – designing a person-centred curriculum framework for educating healthcare professionals.

TABLE 1.4   The Elements of The 7S Framework and Associated Questions.

Element	Questions to guide completion of the 7S system analysis
Strategy	■ What is the curriculum seeking to accomplish? ■ What is distinctive about this curriculum? ■ How does the curriculum adapt to changing healthcare contexts? ■ How has the curriculum been developed through authentic co-design with stakeholders? ■ How is the curriculum structured? ■ What are the reporting and working relationships for delivering the curriculum (hierarchical, flat, siloes, etc.)? ■ How is the team responsible for delivering the curriculum aligned to it? ■ How are decisions about the curriculum made (e.g. is decision making based on centralisation, empowerment, decentralisation or other approaches)? ■ How is information shared (formal and informal channels) across the organisation? ■ How is the learner/stakeholder voice heard in information sharing across the organisation?
Systems	■ What are the primary pedagogical practices that guide the curriculum? ■ What curriculum quality systems and controls are in place? ■ How are the progress and evolution of the curriculum tracked?
Shared values	■ What is the vision of the curriculum and what has shaped its development? ■ What are the stated values of the course team? ■ How do the values influence how the curriculum is delivered? ■ How do the stated curriculum values match those of the stakeholders?
Style	■ What are the management/leadership styles of those responsible for delivering the curriculum? ■ How do team members respond to management/leadership? ■ Do team members function competitively, collaboratively or co-operatively? ■ What behaviours, tasks and deliverables do management/leadership reward?
Staff	■ What are the staffing requirements to deliver the curriculum (e.g. number of staff needed, level of academic preparation, etc.)? ■ Are there gaps in required capabilities or resources?
Skills	■ What skills are needed to deliver the curriculum? Are these skills sufficiently present and available? ■ Are there any skill gaps? ■ What is the department known for doing well? ■ Do the employees have the right capabilities to do their jobs? ■ How are skills monitored and improved?

Designing a Person-centred Curriculum Framework for Educating Healthcare Professionals

In this part of the project, a multiphase, mixed methods design was used to synthesise evidence from multiple sources, to surface the key components of a person-centred curriculum framework. The complete methodology is published elsewhere (O'Donnell et al. 2022). The eight-stage, mixed methods design optimised opportunities for national and transnational collaboration. The eight stages are shown in Figure 1.7

THE CURRICULUM FRAMEWORK

Working from the perspective that while person-centred principles may be context dependent, they are universal and can underpin healthcare education and practice, we present a person-centred curriculum framework (Figure 1.8). Each element of the 7S framework is connected synergistically with the philosophical principles (pragmatism, relationism, co-constructivism and transformation; Dickson et al. 2020) to create healthful, person-centred cultures for education and practice. Ultimately, this results in person-centred practice, brought about by the authentic engagement of stakeholders (educators, practitioners, learners, policy makers) represented at the centre of the model. The coloured spirals represent the 7Ss and the central spirograph represents how all of the four underpinning philosophical principles work together and are woven interconnectedly with the 7Ss.

Strategy

Strategy encompasses the whole curriculum framework that identifies the unique selling point (USP) of the programme and what makes it different, and thus attractive to potential students. In the context of this work, the USP for curriculum development is the explicit and intentional focus on creating person-centred healthcare practitioners. Person-centredness is the aspired standard of healthcare globally but how it is conceptualised and translated across multiple contexts remains a challenge (McCormack 2022). A focus on strategy brings to the fore the requirement for a shared and clear understanding of person-centredness and what this means for programmes, roles and responsibilities. Furthermore, strategy emphasises the importance of a shared language that is meaningful for all persons, including students, educators/academics and practice partners across organisations (Short et al. 2018).

The curriculum framework presented is synergistic with the Person-centred Practice Framework (McCance and McCormack 2021) as a means of making explicit the core concepts that inform the development of competent person-centred healthcare practitioners. The Person-centred Practice Framework, as an underpinning theory for this curriculum framework development project, encapsulates the 7Ss through the core constructs of macro-context, prerequisites and practice environment. Embedded at every level of curriculum design and delivery should be person-centred ways of being that characterise interpersonal relationships and this is consistent with the person-centred processes of the Person-centred Practice Framework. Person-centred ways of

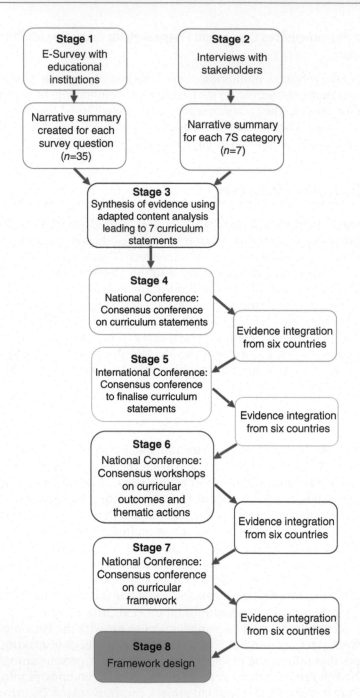

FIGURE 1.7 Overview of methodological stages.

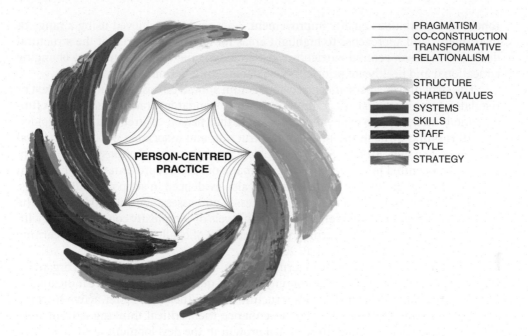

PRAGMATISM
CO-CONSTRUCTION
TRANSFORMATIVE
RELATIONALISM

STRUCTURE
SHARED VALUES
SYSTEMS
SKILLS
STAFF
STYLE
STRATEGY

PERSON-CENTRED
PRACTICE

FIGURE 1.8   The Person-centred Curriculum Framework.

being need to be supported by the strategic goals of the organisation that have person-centredness explicitly stated in their mission/vision/core values and should be 'known' through all layers and parts of the organisation. This strategic embeddedness enables the development of curricula through authentic, collaborative, interdisciplinary partnerships with all stakeholders which, alongside person-centredness, becomes the USP.

The outcomes expected from a curriculum with the strategic foci on person-centredness will embed into and across the curriculum a humanising philosophy that views person-centredness as a way of being; foster person-centred learning cultures where everyone will flourish; and facilitate transformative personal and professional growth as competent and confident person-centred practitioners (Van Schalkwyk et al. 2019).

Structure

In keeping with the strategic drivers, the philosophical principles of person-centredness should be evident in how the curriculum is co-constructed with key stakeholders (Dickson et al. 2020). All stakeholders should be represented, including educators (in academic and practice settings), students, strategy and policy leaders and recipients of healthcare. This could be achieved by establishing an active stakeholder/practice advisory board with the intention of creating collaborative, communicative spaces conducive to authentic co-design, delivery and evaluation (Virgolesi et al. 2020). A partnership approach to curriculum evaluation is also advocated. By triangulating stakeholder perspectives, the evaluation of a person-centred curriculum can support robust and continuous quality improvement. This could be achieved using a range of instruments and approaches to highlight areas for development so that the structural design of a person-centred curriculum remains dynamic and responsive to changing educational and healthcare priorities (Cook et al. 2018; O'Donnell et al. 2020).

The structure of a person-centred curriculum should be designed in the context of regulatory, organisational, programme and quality standards (Franco et al. 2019). A fundamental intention is to explicitly demonstrate that person-centredness is the 'golden thread' running through the programme structure and associated documents (Royal College of Nursing 2012, p. 56). This 'golden thread' can be demonstrated by mapping person-centred principles in a diagrammatic or visual representation to highlight linkages throughout the curriculum that are also evidenced in supporting documents, learning outcomes, unit structures and processes and assessment methodologies. The curriculum structure should reflect increasing levels of complexity commensurate with a constructivist approach to learning where the level of challenge increases as learning occurs (Charles 2018; Dickson et al. 2020).

Affording optimal flexibility in terms of what, when and how learning is organised is aligned with the principles of autonomy and self-determination that are indicative of person-centredness. The curriculum structure should therefore foster active learning and use creativity to inspire learners to enhance their critical thinking and intrinsic motivations for personal and professional growth in the development of their person-centred practice (Bristol et al. 2019).

Systems

Systems that support the development and delivery of a person-centred curriculum should align the teaching, learning and assessment (TLA) methods with the curriculum outcomes, explicitly articulating the philosophical principles of personhood (McCormack and McCance 2017). A person-centred approach reflects the principle of co-construction and requires flexibility; it offers choice for learners and supports them in understanding their own learning needs in relation to person-centred practices (Gaebel et al. 2018; Dickson et al. 2020). Key to person-centred TLA methods are educators and leaders who are committed to embodying the values of person-centredness, using facilitated learning and assessment strategies. They encourage multi-stakeholder assessments and portfolios where learners can use creativity to demonstrate their learning. The systems supporting ownership of learning include developmental tools such as learning analytics to monitor learning and progress. Learners should also have individualised and consistent coaching and mentorship. Creating safe reflective spaces throughout programmes enables learners to explore their personhood (Wald et al. 2019). Facilitated small group reflection gives learners opportunities to explore what is important to them, along with learning from practice. This is fundamental to having cultural humility, whereby learners critically reflect on their values, beliefs and assumptions in the context of shaping their worldview and how they interact with others (Sanchez et al. 2019). Creating spaces for reflection and critical dialogue is core to person-centredness and requires experienced facilitators of learning to help learners make sense of their experiences.

A person-centred curriculum draws explicitly on educational/pedagogical theories that are related to adult (professional) education. Educators are prepared through appropriate programmes and working alongside experienced facilitators, enabling them to find their own style of facilitating learning (Gaebel et al. 2018). They use a range of methods including flipped classrooms, hybrid classroom and opportunities for simulated learning and social learning. They are supported in becoming person-centred facilitators of workplace and work-based learning and assessment and opportunities are created for learners to be immersed in realistic practice environments (such as simulation, living labs, etc.), to enable authentic learning. The curriculum offers multiple/alternative assessment methods that provide choice, while still achieving learning outcomes. Learners should co-design assessments, thereby fostering shared values, understanding and commitment.

Shared Values

A person-centred curriculum is underpinned by shared values that frame the curriculum, by explicitly stating the ethos of the programme. These shared values express the meaning of healthfulness for all stakeholders and focus on the development of learners' personhood and relationships with others, appreciating the uniqueness and potential of all persons. Respecting self-determination and negotiated autonomy are central to a person-centred ethos and there should be an intentional focus on working with, rather than on, persons. Teams, including all stakeholders, should agree specific ways of being person centred in their approaches and attitudes to students and colleagues. They should role model reciprocal respect and understanding in working and learning relationships. According to Hart (2019), it is through authentic interest in the lifeworld of other persons and knowledge of their own lifeworld that team members and recipients of care are able to co-create shared/blended lifeworlds.

The explicitly stated ethos of the programme should enable identification of the agreed expectations and outcomes for all stakeholders. Co-translating discussions will ensure the language of this curriculum framework is meaningful, recognisable and understandable to the various users, and explicitly linked through local policies, documents and concepts (Virgolesi et al. 2020). Conversations are encouraged on the importance of values and creating healthful cultures, i.e. one where decision making is shared, staff relationships are collaborative, leadership is transformational and innovative practices are supported (McCormack and McCance 2017). Other practical ways in which this can be evidenced include making the curriculum ethos explicit in programme documents, including induction and recruitment material; encouraging educators and learners to explicitly acknowledge and discuss the curriculum shared values in, for example, shared stories and role modelling. Other evidence can include creating opportunities for shared decision making and active participation using consensus and/or spaces to create shared purposes and interpretations of a person-centred curriculum (Leal Filho et al. 2018). Curriculum teams can develop a values statement describing what person-centredness could/should mean to everyone (based on and fostering shared meaning and embodiment) and the impact on healthful cultures and its ambassadors.

Shared values should actively embrace challenging viewpoints, role modelling how competing perspectives and peer feedback are managed through different models of dialogical practices. These values are instrumental to enabling embodiment and congruence between what is espoused and behaviours in practice.

Style

Style refers to the style of leadership used to design and deliver the curriculum. Consistent with the philosophical principles of person-centredness, the leadership style should be authentic, collaborative and co-operative (Dickson et al. 2020). This form of transformative leadership is committed to lifelong learning, critical engagement, authentic collaboration, and moral and social purpose (Carey and Coutts 2021). It cultivates diverse thinking and an open sharing of differing perspectives that promote person-centred values and cultures. It is achieved through effective role modelling of person-centredness in leadership practices that foster authentic engagement with students, staff and all stakeholders (O'Donnell 2021).

The leadership style should embrace the principles of collective leadership where all persons are engaged through democratic processes (Raelin 2018). These principles should be explicitly evidenced in quality and governance structures and processes to embed clear expectations about ways of working. In this context, leaders create and support an influential community of ambassadors of person-centredness. Learning needs identify recognition and support for learning, development and transformational change. This approach fosters a shared responsibility for achieving the curriculum outcomes with the aim of humanising healthcare professional learning alongside innovative practices (Al-Husseini et al. 2021). Consistent with the model of person-centred leadership by Cardiff et al. (2018), the approach should foster trust and effectively utilise and develop the talents, expertise and perspectives of all those who contribute to implementation of the curriculum.

Skills

Those designing and delivering a person-centred curriculum should have the ability to collectively create the conditions for learners to flourish in a culture that is underpinned by shared values of person-centredness (Cook 2017; Dollinger et al. 2018). Educators require the knowledge, skills and expertise to be facilitators of person-centred learning, and will use communication and active listening skills to create an environment where learners and educators are seen as partners (O'Donnell 2021). Educators should adopt a leadership style that creates a psychologically safe, open environment where learners can share thoughts and experiences (Brown and McCormack 2016; Wald et al. 2019). A psychologically safe learning environment is achieved by fostering relationships that are collaborative, respectful, reciprocal and inclusive with the shared goal of supporting learners to choose their pathway in a flexible curriculum. Educators provide feedback and feedforward that are timely, transparent and practical. They actively seek feedback through ongoing evaluations and are responsive to it. They draw on self- and peer critique to develop their knowledge skills and expertise (Gómez and Valdés 2019). Educators can recognise and celebrate individual achievements. They have the skills to create the conditions for everyone to flourish in a culture that is underpinned by the shared values of person-centredness (Cook 2017).

For educators to work in these ways, they need to be supported to develop their knowledge, skills and expertise in critical, reflexive and collaborative continuous learning (Sheppard-Law et al. 2018).

Staff

To design, deliver and sustain a person-centred curriculum, all persons involved need to embody values of person-centredness through an explicit commitment to the facilitation of learning. Team capabilities need to be built around staff (leaders and educators) with the necessary knowledge, skills and expertise to facilitate critical, reflexive, collaborative and engaged learning (O'Donnell 2021).

Leaders need to invest in staff development, paying attention to the diversity of team members and their individual learning and development needs. This ensures that the necessary attributes are present for delivering the curriculum (Bruggeman et al. 2020). Leaders should recognise and create opportunities for the staff team to develop their knowledge, skills and expertise in critical, reflexive, collaborative learning, for example through induction, peer supported activities, sharing best practice, curriculum design initiation events and curriculum evaluation workshops. Critical reflexive learning, peer learning and mentorship provide other ways of facilitating the development of person-centred staff (Manley et al. 2013). These practices facilitate staff to articulate and illustrate the meaning of person-centredness for professional practice, curriculum development and delivery. Psychologically safe spaces underpin the delivery of safe spaces for collaborative learning (Turner and Harder 2018). Leaders need to be attentive to optimum staff/student ratios and diversity of skills to realise effective teaching, with facilitation being at the heart of TLA practices.

CONCLUSION

In this chapter we have introduced the comprehensive collaborative research and development work we undertook to develop the first Universal Curriculum Framework for Person-centred Healthcare Practitioner Education. Our motivation for undertaking this work is to challenge the status quo, raise consciousness and stimulate action to help everyone in healthcare think about how best to provide person-centred healthcare to persons, people and populations. Any curriculum that purports to focus on a person-centred philosophy needs to extend beyond 'understanding person-centredness' to helping all practitioners develop the knowledge, skills and expertise in creating the kinds of workplace cultures where all persons can flourish.

This is clearly not the responsibility of any one practitioner or indeed any one profession. Instead, it requires engagement of all professionals, all layers of organisational governance and leadership and all parts of complex organisational systems. We have tried to reflect this complexity in our proposed curriculum framework. However, we do not see it as a recipe but rather as a heuristic device that can help teams engage in critical discussions about curriculum content, the systems needed to enable meaningful learning and the cultures required to facilitate effective learning and development. We have not limited the idea of 'curriculum' to learning that happens in formal education institutions but consider the framework as being applicable to programmes of learning that happen throughout the health system. This principle that learning how to be an effective person-centred practitioner happens in all parts of the healthcare ecology is critical to the way in which the remainder of this book is structured.

OVERVIEW OF THE BOOK

The remaining chapters of this book take you through each of the seven components of the curriculum framework – the 7S framework. In Chapter 2 we begin with addressing strategy. Just as we position person-centred practice in a macro healthcare context, we also need to position curricula in the strategic contexts in which they exist. A curriculum addresses the key strategic agendas it aims to connect with, as well as being a strategy in and of itself for advancing the requisite knowledge, skills and expertise needed for developing person-centred practices in healthcare settings. We view curriculum as a whole system as reflected in our definition of a 'shared curriculum framework'.

Having considered the strategic framework of the curriculum, in Chapter 3 we then turn to the curriculum structures. All curricula adhere to particular structures, some of which are determined by professional body regulatory frameworks and specific university regulations. When we consider structures in a person-centred curriculum, we include these predetermined structures while at the same time paying attention to how we structure curricula to maximise person-centredness in all aspects of teaching, learning and facilitation engagements.

In Chapter 4 we address the systems needed to operationalise a person-centred curriculum. We consider all aspects of an educational system necessary to work in a person-centred way and that enable person-centred learning to occur. The need for coherent and relevant learning theories is addressed and for these to reinforce person-centred principles and practices.

Without a clear set of shared values, we know that a person-centred curriculum cannot be sustained. Person-centred values are key to the being, doing and becoming of learners who are developing as person-centred practitioners. In Chapter 5 we explore the shared values that are central to the person-centred curriculum framework.

Chapter 6 considers the importance of leadership style in curriculum development, implementation and delivery. There is a growing evidence base supporting the importance of person-centred leadership and its importance in facilitating the development of person-centredness, whatever the context. We advocate for distributive models of leadership that generate collective responsibility and accountability for curriculum processes and outcomes.

In Chapter 7 we address the staff attributes and qualities needed to enable the facilitation of a person-centred learning culture. Staff development is critical in this context and we consider the continuous development of 'self' as an essential commitment to a culture of shared learning for all. Even with excellent person-centred leadership, without a staff team that is committed to working with the agreed shared values and to the flourishing of learners, the outcomes of a person-centred curriculum cannot be achieved.

Chapter 8 continues the people focus and considers the skills needed to work in a person-centred way when facilitating learning and development. We know that didactic models of teaching, for example, have limited impact when considering person-centred ways of learning and so we explore the range of skills needed to alter our practices as person-centred educators and facilitators of learning and development.

Finally in Chapter 9 we provide a range of examples of person-centred curriculum in action. We draw on the collective knowledge, skills and experience of the authors to present a variety of stories about our experiences of implementing person-centred curricula. We do not intend these to be 'ideal models' or 'perfect examples' but we do hope that they help to bring to life different aspects of the curriculum framework and provide further insights into how these parts of the framework could work in practice – warts and all!!

Throughout the book, we provide tools, methods and processes you can draw upon to implement the Person-centred Curriculum Framework in your context. We engage in reflective dialogue with you, the reader, and guide you in using these activities so you can capitalise on your potential for successful implementation. We know you will have a range of other tools, methods and resources that you can draw up and we encourage you to do so. We would be delighted if you can share these with others engaged in person-centred curriculum development and implementation so that we can continue to grow this global community of learning facilitators and educators committed to advancing person-centred healthcare.

REFERENCES

Al-Husseini, S., El Beltagi, I., and Moizer, J. (2021). Transformational leadership and innovation: the mediating role of knowledge sharing amongst higher education faculty. *International Journal of Leadership in Education* 24 (5): 670–693.

Boomer, C. and McCormack, B. (2010). Creating the conditions for growth: a collaborative practice development programme for clinical nurse leaders. *Journal of Advanced Nursing* 18 (6): 633–644.

Bristol, T., Hagler, D., McMillian-Bohler, J. et al. (2019). Nurse educators' use of lecture and active learning. *Teaching and Learning in Nursing* 14 (2): 94–96.

Brown, D. and McCormack, B. (2016). Exploring psychological safety as a component of facilitation within the promoting action research in health services framework. *Journal of Clinical Nursing* 25 (19–20): 2912–2932.

Bruggeman, B., Tondeur, J., Struyven, K. et al. (2020). Experts speaking: crucial teacher attributes for implementing blended learning in higher education. *The Internet and Higher Education*. 48.

Cardiff, S., McCormack, B., and McCance, T. (2018). Person-centred leadership: a relational approach to leadership derived through action research. *Journal of Clinical Nursing* 27 (15–16): 3056–3069.

Carey, G. and Coutts, L. (2021). Fostering transformative professionalism through curriculum changes within a bachelor of music. In: *Expanding Professionalism in Music and Higher Music Education* (ed. H. Westerlund and H. Gaunt), 42–58. Oxford: Routledge.

Charles, A. (2018). Rivers and fireworks: social constructivism in education. In: *Dynamic Learning Spaces in Education* (ed. V. Kapur and S. Ghose), 285–300. Singapore: Springer.

Cook, N. (2017). Co-creating Person-centred Learning and Development Experiences with Student Nurses in Practice through Action Research. Doctoral dissertation, Ulster University.

Cook, N., McCance, T., McCormack, B. et al. (2018). Perceived caring attributes and priorities of preregistration nursing students throughout a nursing curriculum underpinned by person-centredness. *Journal of Clinical Nursing* 27 (13–14): 2847–2858.

Dickson, C., van Lieshout, F., Kmetec, S. et al. (2020). Developing philosophical and pedagogical principles for a pan-European person-centred curriculum framework. *International Practice Development Journal* 10 (Suppl 2): 1–20.

Dollinger, M., Lodge, J., and Coates, H. (2018). Co-creation in higher education: towards a conceptual model. *Journal of Marketing for Higher Education* 28 (2): 210–231.

Franco, I., Saito, O., Vaughter, P. et al. (2019). Higher education for sustainable development: actioning the global goals in policy, curriculum and practice. *Sustainability Science* 14 (6): 1621–1642.

Gadamer, H. and Dutt, C. (1993). *Hermeneutik, Ästhetik, Praktische Philosophie: Hans-Georg Gadamer im Gespräch [Hermeneutics, Aesthetics, Practical Philosophy: An Interview with Hans-Georg Gadamer]*. Winter, Germany: Universitätsverlag C. Winter.

Gaebel, M., Zhang, T., Bunescu, L., and Stoeber, H. (2018). *Learning and Teaching in the European Higher Education Area*. Brussels: European University Association.

Gómez, L. and Valdés, M. (2019). The evaluation of teacher performance in higher education. *Propositos y Representaciones. Revista de Psicología Educativa* 7 (2): 499–515.

Hart, W. (2019). *Lost in Control: Re-focus on Purpose*. Rosmalen, The Netherlands: Verdraaide Organisaties.

Heidegger, M. (1967). *Being and Time*. Oxford: Blackwell.

Leal Filho, W., Raath, S., Lazzarini, B. et al. (2018). The role of transformation in learning and education for sustainability. *Journal of Cleaner Production* 199: 286–295.

Manley, K., Titchen, A., and McCormack, B. (2013). What is practice development and what are the starting points? In: *Practice Development in Nursing and Healthcare*, 2e (ed. B. McCormack, K. Manley, and A. Titchen), 45–65. Oxford: Wiley-Blackwell.

McCance, T. and McCormack, B. (2021). The person-centred practice framework. In: *Fundamentals of Person-Centred Healthcare Practice* (ed. B. McCormack, T. McCance, S. Martin, et al.), 23–32. Oxford: Wiley.

McCormack, B. (2022). Person-centred care and measurement: the more one sees, the better one knows where to look. *Journal of Health Services Research & Policy* 27 (2): 85–87.

McCormack, B. and Dewing, J. (2019). International Community of Practice for person-centred practice: position statement on person-centredness in health and social care. *International Practice Development Journal* 9 (1): 1–7.

McCormack, B., Magowan, R., O'Donnell, D., Phelan, A., Štiglic, G. and van Lieshout, F. (2022) Developing a Person-centred Curriculum Framework: a whole-systems methodology. International Practice Development Journal. Vol 12, Special Issue, Article 2 https://doi.org/10.19043/ipdj.12suppl.002

McCormack, B. and McCance, T. (ed.) (2017). *Person-Centred Practice in Nursing and Health Care: Theory and Practice*. Chichester: Wiley Blackwell.

McCormack, B., McCance. TV., Martin, S. (2021). What is Person-centredness. In: *Fundamentals of Person-Centred Healthcare Practice* (eds. McCormack B, McCance T, Martin S, McMillan A, Bulley C), 19, Oxford: Wiley.

O'Donnell, D. (2021). Becoming a Person-centred Healthcare Professional: A Mixed Methods Study. Doctoral thesis, Ulster University.

O'Donnell, D., McCormack, B., McCance, T., and McIlfatrick, S. (2020). A meta-synthesis of personcentredness in nursing curricula. *International Practice Development Journal* 10 (Suppl 2): 1–22.

O'Donnell, D., Dickson, C., Phelan, A. et al. (2022). A mixed methods approach to the development of a person-centred curriculum framework: surfacing person-centred principles and practices. *International Practice Development Journal* 12 (Suppl): 1–14.

Phelan, A., McCormack, B., Dewing, J. et al. (2020). Review of developments in person-centred healthcare. *International Practice Development Journal*. 10: Special issue.

Raelin, J. (2018). What are you afraid of: collective leadership and its learning implications. *Management Learning* 49 (1): 59–66.

Royal College of Nursing (2012). *Quality with Compassion: The Future of Nursing Education*. London: Royal College of Nursing.

Sanchez, N., Norka, A., Corbin, M., and Peters, C. (2019). Use of experiential learning, reflective writing, and metacognition to develop cultural humility among undergraduate students. *Journal of Social Work Education* 55 (1): 75–88.

van Schalkwyk, S.C., Hafler, J., Brewer, T. et al. (2019). Transformative learning as pedagogy for the health professions: a scoping review. *Medical Education* 53 (6): 547–558.

Sheppard-Law, S., Curtis, S., Bancroft, J. et al. (2018). Novice clinical nurse educator's experience of a self-directed learning, education and mentoring program: a qualitative study. *Contemporary Nurse* 54 (2): 208–219.

Short, M., Dempsey, K., Ackland, J. et al. (2018). What is a person? Deepening students' and colleagues' understanding of person-centredness. *Advances in Social Work and Welfare Education*. 20 (1): 139–156.

Turner, S. and Harder, N. (2018). Psychological safe environment: a concept analysis. *Clinical Simulation in Nursing* 18: 47–55.

Virgolesi, M., Marchetti, A., Pucciarelli, G. et al. (2020). Stakeholders' perspective about their engagement in developing a competency-based nursing baccalaureate curriculum: a qualitative study. *Journal of Professional Nursing* 36 (3): 141–146.

Wald, H., White, J., Reis, S. et al. (2019). Grappling with complexity: medical students' reflective writings about challenging patient encounters as a window into professional identity formation. *Medical Teacher* 41 (2): 152–160.

Waterman, J., Peters, T., and Phillips, J. (1980). Structure is not organization. *Business Horizons* 23 (3): 14–26.

CHAPTER 2

Strategy

In this chapter we work with you to explore ideas around 'strategy' in person-centred curricula and ways in which strategy shapes the way that the curriculum is positioned in your programme of work. We are very aware that strategy can seem a bit daunting and 'distant' from our everyday reality of practice, so in this chapter we want to engage with you from the perspective of strategy as a practical tool for shaping your decisions when designing your curriculum, whatever your context. We will work with key elements of strategy and offer methods, tools and approaches to bring these elements to life in your work. There is no prescription for designing or working with strategy, but adopting a systematic approach to developing, analysing and implementing strategy is important as you will hopefully see as we move through this resource – we say that because many of the elements of strategy that we explore in this chapter will be revisited as we move through other chapters. The methods, tools and approaches we offer here are not exhaustive and you may have others that you are familiar with and are helpful to you also.

INTRODUCTION

This chapter focuses on the strategy component of the Person-centred Curriculum Framework. In this framework, we define strategy as:

> the whole curriculum framework that identifies the unique selling point (USP) of the programme and what makes it unique, and thus attractive to potential students.

A person-centred curriculum has the explicit and intentional focus on developing person-centred healthcare practitioners. Person-centredness is the aspired-to standard of healthcare globally; however, how it is conceptualised and translated across

Developing Person-Centred Cultures in Healthcare Education and Practice: An Essential Guide, First Edition.
Edited by Brendan McCormack.
© 2024 John Wiley & Sons Ltd. Published 2024 by John Wiley & Sons Ltd.

multiple contexts remains a challenge (McCormack 2022). A focus on strategy brings to the fore the requirement for a shared and clear common understanding of person-centredness and what this means for education programmes, roles and responsibilities. Furthermore, strategy emphasises the importance of a shared language that is meaningful for all persons, including students, educators and practice partners across organisations (Carvalho et al. 2021). The Person-centred Curriculum Framework is synergistic with the Person-centred Practice Framework (McCance and McCormack 2021) as a means of making explicit the core concepts that inform the development of competent person-centred healthcare practitioners.

Person-centred ways of being must be supported by the strategic goals of the organisation that have person-centredness explicitly stated in their core values, mission statement and vision, and should be 'known' through all layers and parts of the organisation. This strategic embeddedness enables the development of curricula through authentic, collaborative, interdisciplinary partnerships with all stakeholders which, alongside person-centredness, becomes its USP.

The outcomes expected from a curriculum with the strategic focus of person-centredness will:

- embed a humanising philosophy that views person-centredness as a way of being into and across the curriculum
- foster person-centred learning cultures where everyone will flourish, and facilitate transformative personal and professional growth as competent and confident person-centred practitioners (Van Schalkwyk et al. 2019).

Within our definition of strategy, we identify three strategic foci of a person-centred curriculum.

1. Developing person-centred learning cultures.
2. Developing competent and confident person-centred practitioners.
3. Developing flourishing cultures that nurture authentic professional and therapeutic relationships.

This strategic focus is embedded in a humanising philosophy that views person-centredness as a way of being.

ACTIVITY 2.1

You probably have access to an existing curriculum in your team, unit, school, faculty or organisation that is used for the education of healthcare practitioners. Have a look at the curriculum and consider how explicit these three purposes are in that curriculum. You might like to make some reflective notes as you progress through the activity so you can revisit them in later chapters.

1. What does the curriculum say about the type of learning culture being promoted?
2. Is it person centred? In what way(s) is it person centred?

3. What does the curriculum say about the kind of practitioners being developed?
4. Is a holistic approach to practice advocated? You might like to read the article by Rotthoff et al. (2021) on holistic assessment of competence and where the idea of competence as holistic practice is explored.
5. You might also like to read the paper by Dickson et al. (2020) and consider how the espoused philosophical and methodological principles relate to the curriculum you are reviewing: www.fons.org/library/journal/volume10-suppl2/article4. What critical questions does it raise for you?

In undertaking this activity, you may have uncovered or revealed some taken-for-granted assumptions embedded in the curriculum. Sometimes curricula are 'silent' about the type of learning culture that is valued, but it is made visible implicitly through the privileged approaches to learning that are set out in units of study, teaching and learning methods and assessment methods. While the practitioner of the future may be espoused in the curriculum philosophy (for example), you might have found that there is little to show what that means in detail, or that it is assumed to be visible through stated learning outcomes. In these situations, person-centredness is left to 'chance' and open to multiple interpretations by those delivering the curriculum content. If you had a chance to read the paper by Dickson et al., you will have noted the emphasis we place on having an explicit and clearly articulated philosophical perspective, so that content is consistent and clear in terms of how all practices systematically work towards developing person-centred healthcare practitioners.

Arising from the three strategic foci introduced above, collaborators in the development of the Person-centred Curriculum Framework identified a range of thematic actions that should be considered when strategically positioning a person-centred curriculum. These actions will shape the content of much of this chapter as we progress through it together.

Thematic Actions

1. Promote person-centredness being explicitly stated in the organisational core values, mission statement and vision.
2. Foster a shared clear understanding of person-centredness and what this means for programmes, roles and responsibilities (operationalisation into other Ss).
3. Adopt authentic, collaborative, interdisciplinary development of curricula in partnership with all stakeholders which, alongside person-centredness, becomes the unique selling point for the outside world.
4. Consider adapting and translating the language of the Person-centred Curriculum Framework to ensure that the various users (academic, stakeholder and student perspectives) are recognisable and understandable for all.

FREQUENTLY ASKED QUESTIONS ABOUT STRATEGY

What is Strategy?

Strategy is a high-level perspective of the organisation. It sets out how to enhance the success of the organisation's work through capitalising on its unique value. It encompasses the conditions of possibility for success in achieving its mission and shared vision, something we will address later in this chapter. This is achieved by the articulation of activities which the organisation uses to realise its objectives and is mindful of planning in response to or anticipation of change to retain customers and increase market share (Waterman et al. 1980, p. 20). So strategic planning needs to encompass aspects of sustainability that are underpinned by the organisation's values and mission (Odeh 2021). Thus, the organisation itself can be a source of strength or weakness.

What is Strategy in a Curriculum?

Within curricula, strategy is immersed in areas of teaching used to enable learners to navigate the professional competencies to be demonstrated, as well as making explicit ways in which learners and staff experience theoretical and applied aspects of the programme.

Why is Strategy Important in Curricula?

The importance of strategy is underpinned by its focus on providing the direction of the organisation's aims and establishing the exclusive selling point being striven for. It needs to be dynamic and evolve with and adapt to future contexts in a dynamic way. Typically, learning environments in a university or healthcare organisation will have developed mission statements, shared vision, philosophies of learning/practice, learning aims and objectives that will direct the context of learning and development.

Here we provide an example of an agreed shared vision, values and commitments that underpin a strategic plan (presented as an integrated mandala) developed by the Susan Wakil School of Nursing and Midwifery at the University of Sydney.

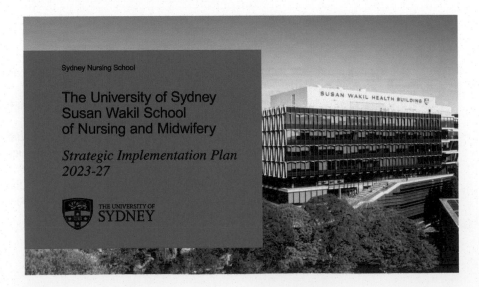

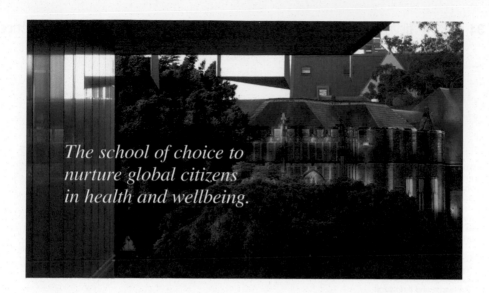

*The school of choice to
nurture global citizens
in health and wellbeing.*

Vision, Values and Commitments

Through our creative and collaborative discussions and engagement with key stakeholders, we identified **five core values** to guide or ways of being and doing in Sydney Nursing School and **five commitments** that we make to each other to work towards creating an effective workplace culture and developing respectful and productive relationships locally, nationally and globally.

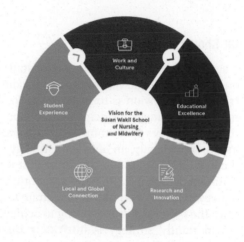

Vision, Values and Commitments

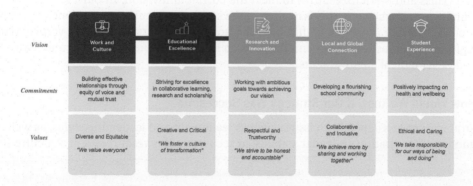

	Work and Culture	Educational Excellence	Research and Innovation	Local and Global Connection	Student Experience
Vision	Work and Culture	Educational Excellence	Research and Innovation	Local and Global Connection	Student Experience
Commitments	Building effective relationships through equity of voice and mutual trust	Striving for excellence in collaborative learning, research and scholarship	Working with ambitious goals towards achieving our vision	Developing a flourishing school community	Positively impacting on health and wellbeing
Values	Diverse and Equitable *"We value everyone"*	Creative and Critical *"We foster a culture of transformation"*	Respectful and Trustworthy *"We strive to be honest and accountable"*	Collaborative and Inclusive *"We achieve more by sharing and working together"*	Ethical and Caring *"We take responsibility for our ways of being and doing"*

Action and development plan

We have the opportunity to build on our record of innovation and leadership in nursing and health by enabling all those who engage with us to benefit from the world-leading resources of the school, the wider faculty and the university.

We are committed to striving for excellence in collaborative learning, research and scholarship and to working with ambitious goals towards achieving our vision.

We will do this through five focused strategic areas:
- Work and culture
- Educational excellence
- Research and Innovation
- Local and global connection
- Student experience

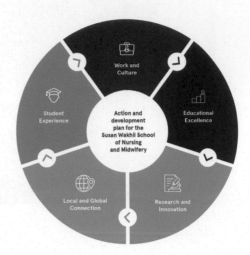

What Should a Strategy Include?

The strategy should be inspirational for staff and students and explicitly state goals that align with the strategic vision, enabling a competitive advantage. With a person-centred curriculum, the vision is to foster a supportive partnership in learning and development that encourages principles of collaboration, democratic learning and curiosity within experiences that embrace the diversity of the community of learners and co-learners. Accordingly, an optimum strategy is clearly articulated, monitored over time and can be time-limited in the sense that it responds to issues of service need, policy orientation, learning approaches and regulatory demands. Essentially, the elements of a strategy, taken as a whole, demonstrate to everyone who engages with it the kind of culture the organisation is aspiring to achieve.

Importantly, strategy is intricately interlinked with the other elements of the Person-centred Curriculum Framework as applied to the learning and development environment. Consequently, the key to using the framework is establishing 'strategic fit'. What we mean by that is the balancing of strategy in terms of it being embedded in and co-ordinated with the other elements of the curriculum, so as to assure success. Strategy employs a compelling direction, a strong structure and a supportive context (Hass and Mortensen 2016) to meet the curriculum vision. In our Person-centred Curriculum Framework, this is explicit in the systems and cultures components, which include learning processes within both the horizontal (hierarchical) and vertical (collegial) systems, as well as an emphasis on collaborations within systems and learning and development environments.

How Would We Know If Our Strategy Was Successful?

Strategic success depends on issues such as leadership and leadership styles, as well as good communication. A leader's ability to secure process resources and structure the curriculum's delivery accordingly while motivating educators and students to pursue the vision is a critical factor. Analysing strategy can identify the position of support (or not) in the total learning experience and expose the need to reframe or change other aspects of the curriculum framework.

Waterman et al. (1980, p. 15) note that strategy is concerned with 'getting it done' and carefully planned strategies may fail due to issues with execution and a lack of attention to all parts of the Person-centred Curriculum Framework. In education, this translates into pragmatic and realistic endeavours to critically identify the most effective way to meet strategic goals. However, this is not a simple task, as executing a strategy, no matter how brilliant, requires the tools for implementation. Because organisations are unique, what is achieved in one learning environment may not be transferable to another. Equally, as curricula for healthcare professions straddle academic and clinical environments, the goal is strategy alignment in both intra- and inter-learning and development environments. Success is based on finding 'a good doable strategy' (Peters and Warterman 1982) that transcends the simplicity of depending on structures to drive implementation, to a position where culture is the driving force in translating the Person-centred Curriculum Framework into everyday practice.

UNPACKING THE STRATEGIC THEMES

Earlier, we identified the four strategic action themes that we synthesised from the many suggestions provided by project collaborators. Essentially these themes enable a strategy to come alive, to turn it from a statement of intent to something that is living in everyday practice, informing and being informed by the other parts of the person-centred curriculum and guiding practice in a systematic way. Essentially, these four themes can be summarised into the following four areas of activity.

- Developing, exploring and engaging a person-centred stance.
- Exploring existing culture and context.
- Developing a shared vision and mission.
- Engaging authentically and meaningfully.

In this section we unpack these strategic action themes and provide processes, tools and methods that can help bring a curriculum strategy to life.

Developing a Person-centred Stance

Person-centredness is a global movement in healthcare simply because it reflects the importance of keeping people at the centre of healthcare systems. It prioritises the human experience and places compassion, dignity and humanistic caring principles at the centre of planning and decision making and is translated through relationships that are built on effective interpersonal processes. We advocate the importance of the underpinning values of person-centredness, where the core value of 'respect for the person' is paramount.

Social models of health recognise that our health is influenced by a wide range of individual, interpersonal, organisational, social, environmental, political and economic factors. This encourages us to have a deeper understanding of health. We have argued that healthfulness is *the* outcome arising from the development of person-centred workplace cultures. Healthfulness (reflecting the idea of promoting good health) is not a concept that is generally used in the healthcare arena. This idea of promoting good health is a necessary but insufficient condition for person-centred practice. Healthfulness means ensuring that the environment in which healthcare is experienced places individual health and well-being of all persons as the core concern. For healthful cultures to be achieved, all persons need to be energised by the context in which they work and for that energy to connect with the personhood of all persons. This perspective on well-being ensures that person-centredness is not a unidirectional activity focusing on ensuring that service users have a good care experience at the expense of staff well-being.

There are challenges within healthcare systems that affect the development of healthful workplace cultures. A shared language is essential if we are to bring about system-wide change. While person-centredness permeates healthcare strategy and policy, the reality is that often stakeholders are not talking about the same thing. We also see this dilemma in the published literature, with interchangeable use of terms such as family centred, patient centred, people centred and relationship centred, leading to arguments that person-centredness is 'too difficult to define' (Klancnik Gruden et al. 2020). Furthermore, we see this very issue reflected in the campaigns calling for a refocusing on compassion, caring and kindness. While these are important values within healthcare systems, the challenge is how they manifest in our and other people's behaviours and the influence of attitudinal and moral factors. A shared language is the foundation that supports the development of a shared understanding of person-centred practice and the issues that need to be addressed to bring about sustainable change.

At a level of principle, the understanding of person-centredness is well rehearsed and involves treating people as individuals, respecting their rights as a person, building mutual trust and understanding, and developing therapeutic relationships. Central to this is our explicit focus on all people as persons and the promotion of workplace cultures that promote the well-being of those delivering care as well as those receiving care. This shared understanding, however, needs to be more than an emphasis on the commonly agreed principles that underpin person-centredness. There needs to be an understanding of how these principles can be implemented in practice to bring about positive outcomes, that being the development of healthful cultures that enables flourishing for all.

The Person-centred Curriculum Framework has as its point of departure the Person-centred Practice Framework of McCormack and McCance (2017). This is a theoretical model developed from practice, for use in practice. The Person-centred Practice Framework has evolved over two decades of research and development activity and has made a significant contribution to the landscape of person-centredness globally. Not only does it enable articulation of the dynamic nature of person-centredness, recognising complexity at different levels within healthcare systems, but it offers a common language and a shared understanding of person-centred practice to guide clinical practice, leadership, learning, research and quality improvement. The Person-centred Practice Framework is underpinned by the following definition of person-centredness:

> An approach to practice established through the formation and fostering of healthful relationships between all care providers, service users and others significant to them in their lives. It is underpinned by values of respect for persons, individual right to self-determination, mutual respect and understanding. It is enabled by cultures of empowerment that foster continuous approaches to practice development.
>
> *(McCormack and McCance 2017, p. 3)*

The Person-centred Practice Framework comprises five domains.

- *Prerequisites*, which focus on the attributes of staff.
- The *practice environment*, which focuses on the context in which healthcare is experienced.
- The *person-centred processes*, which focus on ways of engaging that are necessary to create connections between persons.
- The *outcome*, which is the result of effective person-centred practice.
- Finally, these domains sit within the broader *macro-context* (the fifth domain), reflecting factors which are strategic and political in nature that influence the development of person-centred cultures.

The relationships between the five domains of the Person-centred Practice Framework are represented pictorially in Figure 2.1, so that to reach the centre of the framework, one must first take account of the macro-context, followed by consideration of the attributes of staff, as a prerequisite to managing the practice environment and engaging effectively through the person-centred processes. This ordering ultimately leads to the achievement of the outcome – the central component of the framework. It is also important to recognise that there are relationships and overlap between the constructs within each domain.

The *macro-context* reflects the strategic and political factors that influence the development of person-centred cultures. These factors operate regionally (within country), nationally, internationally and globally. The World Health Organization (WHO 2007), Institute for Healthcare Improvement People and Family-centred Care Programme (www.ihi.org/Topics/PFCC/Pages/default.aspx) and Health Foundation (2016) have each produced strategic frameworks for developing health systems that draw on principles of integration, population health promotion and illness prevention as well as 'people-centred' approaches to healthcare delivery. Alongside these international and global strategic frameworks, many of the principles outlined have been translated into national policies and strategies that guide, inform and regulate healthcare delivery; for example, it is common practice these days for professional codes of conduct to include statements and standards for person-centred care and practice or for national strategy documents to be located within a person-centred healthcare frame of reference – for example the values expressed by the Nursing and Midwifery Board of Ireland (www.nmbi.ie/NMBI/media/NMBI/Position-Paper-Values-for-Nurses-and-Midwives-June-2016.pdf).

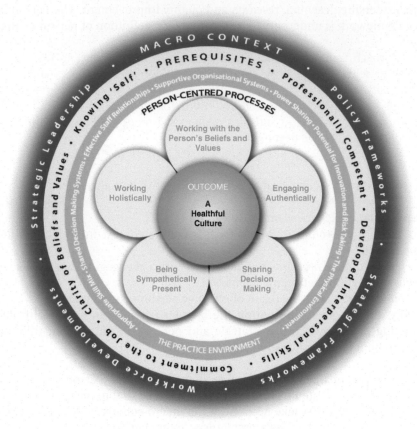

FIGURE 2.1   Person-centred practice framework.

Regionally, these national strategies are translated into strategic plans, strategic goals and key performance indicators of healthcare delivery organisations and their funders. Attributes of the macro-context include policy frameworks, strategic frameworks, workforce developments, and strategic leadership (Figure 2.2).

The *prerequisites* focus on the attributes of staff and are key building blocks in the development of healthcare workers who can deliver effective person-centred care. Attributes include being professionally competent, having developed interpersonal skills, being committed to the job, being able to demonstrate clarity of beliefs and values, and knowing self. There is no hierarchy in relation to these attributes, with all considered of equal importance, but it is the combination of attributes that reflects a person-centred individual who can manage the challenges of a constantly changing context (Figure 2.3).

The *practice environment* reflects the complexity of the context in which healthcare is experienced. The position taken within the Person-centred Practice Framework is that context is synonymous with the practice environment, and contained within it are multifaceted characteristics and qualities of the environment (people, processes and structures) that affect the effectiveness of person-centred practice. To this end,

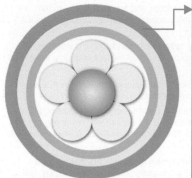

Health & social care/policy: the decisions, plans, and actions that are undertaken to achieve specific health and social care goals within a society (adapted from WHO https://www.who.int/health-topics/health-systems-governance//tab tab 1)

Strategic frameworks: an aspirational roadmap that presents the relationships between and within an organisation's strategic goals and the programmes of work to achieve those goals

Workforce developments: a wide range of activities, policies and programmes employed to create, sustain, and retain a viable workforce that can provide current and future healthcare

Strategic leadership: a practice in which executive leaders develop a vision, and use different styles of management, leadership and influence, to help organisations and teams to adapt so as to remain efficient and effective in a changing economic and technological climate

FIGURE 2.2 Defining the macro-context.

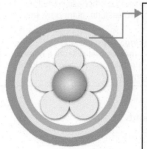

Professionally competent: the knowledge, skills and attitudes of the person to negotiate care options, and effectively provide holistic care

Developed interpersonal skills: the ability of the person to communicate at a variety of levels with others, using effective verbal and non-verbal interactions that show personal concern for their situation and a commitment to finding mutual solutions

Knowing self: the way a person makes sense of his/her knowing, being and becoming through reflection, self-awareness, and engagement with others

Clarity of belief and values: awareness of the impact of beliefs and values on the healthcare experience and the commitment to reconciling beliefs and values in ways that facilitate person-centredness

Commitment to the job: demonstrated commitment of persons through intentional engagement that focuses on achieving the best possible outcomes

FIGURE 2.3 Defining the prerequisites.

seven characteristics of the care environment are described within the framework: appropriate skill mix; systems that facilitate shared decision making; sharing of power; effective staff relationships; organisational systems that are supportive; potential for innovation and risk taking; and the physical environment. Furthermore, we would contend that the constructs that comprise the practice environment have a significant impact on the operationalisation of person-centred practice and have the greatest potential to limit or enhance the facilitation of person-centred processes (Figure 2.4).

Person-centred processes focus on ways of engaging that are necessary to create connections between persons, which include working with the person's beliefs and values; engaging authentically; being sympathetically present; sharing decision making; and working holistically. In the Person-centred Practice Framework, the person-centred processes apply to all those involved in healthcare delivery and those in receipt of care. It is important at the outset to acknowledge that the person-centred processes are synergistic and often interwoven in the delivery of healthcare (Figure 2.5).

The expected *outcome* to arise from the development of effective person-centred practice is a healthful culture. A healthful culture is one in which decision making is shared, relationships are collaborative, leadership is transformational and innovative

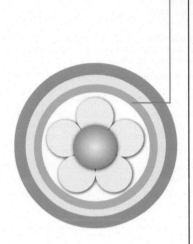

Appropriate skill mix: the number and range of staff with the requisite knowledge and skills needed to provide a quality service relevant to the context

Shared decision-making systems: organisational commitment to collaborative, inclusive and participative ways of engaging within and between teams

Effective staff relationships: interpersonal connections that are productive in the achievement of holistic person-centred care

Power sharing: Non-dominant, non-hierarchical relationships that do not exploit people, but instead are concerned with achieving the best mutually agreed outcomes through agreed values, goals, wishes and desires

Physical environment: healthcare environments that balance aesthetics with function by paying attention to design, dignity, privacy, sanctuary, choice/control, safety, and universal access with the intention of improving patient, family and staff operational performance and outcomes (adapted from HfH 2008)

Supportive organisational systems: organisational systems that promote initiative, creativity, freedom and safety of persons, underpinned by a governance framework that emphasises culture, relationships, values, communication, professional autonomy, and accountability

Potential for innovation and risk taking: the exercising of professional accountability in decision-making that reflects a balance between the best available evidence, professional judgement, local information, and patient/family preferences

FIGURE 2.4   Defining the characteristics of the practice environment.

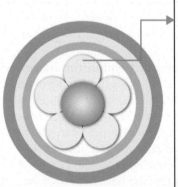

Working with the person's beliefs and values: having a clear picture of what the person's values about his/her life and how he/she makes sense of what is happening from their individual perspective, psychosocial context and social role

Shared decision-making: engaging persons in decision-making by considering values, experiences, concerns and future aspirations

Engaging authentically: the connectedness between people, determined by knowledge of the person, clarity of beliefs and values, knowledge of self and professional expertise

Being sympathetically present: an engagement that recognises the uniqueness and value of the person, by appropriately responding to cues that maximise coping resources through the recognition of important agendas in their life

Working holistically: ways of connecting that pay attention to the whole person through the integration of physiological, psychological, sociocultural, developmental and spiritual dimensions of persons

FIGURE 2.5   Defining the person-centred processes.

practices are supported. Development of a healthful culture has the potential to create conditions that enable human flourishing for those who give care and those who receive care.

Person-centred practice, when understood as a concept embedded in every strategy and policy, has the potential to shape healthcare planning and delivery.

The Person-centred Practice Framework is inclusive of all persons, and it clearly articulates how key components can be embedded in everyday practices at macro-, meso- and micro-levels of practice, with the ultimate outcome of developing a workplace that enables human flourishing for all.

The Person-centred Curriculum Framework translates these domains and constructs into curricula. While the Person-centred Practice Framework is healthcare practice focused, we know the same principles apply in the context of learning and development. By drawing on the philosophical framework, learning methodologies and methods that shape the Person-centred Curriculum Framework, the constructs of the Person-centred Practice Framework are brought to life and embedded in how learning and development are facilitated. This creates a synergy between learning, development and everyday practice, while increasing the potential for person-centred practice cultures to be sustained long-term.

> The transformation of silence into language and action is an act of self-revelation.
>
> *(Lorde 1977)*

This overview of person-centredness as a 'stance' can rightly be considered an idealised vision that might seem unachievable and a reality that is hard to imagine. But we know it can and does exist and that these kinds of cultures are powerful places for all to realise their potential as persons. However, we also know that often what is talked about is far from the reality of what happens. We know that one of the hardest things for any of us to recognise is that we might not be as person centred as we think we are or tell others we are! We sometimes have a 'blind spot' when it comes to our own ways of being and doing and it is easier to notice others and their ways of being and doing, so being reflective is essential to being person centred. Throughout this book, the importance of reflection is highlighted and so you will see reference to reflection and a range of reflective activities throughout each chapter. This is important as the Person-centred Curriculum Framework sees person-centredness as the 'golden thread' of the framework and we need to continuously reflect on each part of it and ensure we are not losing sight of person-centredness in the framework as we go through its implementation.

But we have all probably had the experience of listening to someone talk about their practice and thinking 'That is not how I have seen you practise' or 'Do you actually know what person-centred practice is?' ... or a range of similar thoughts. Often, we are unaware of the disconnect or incongruity between what we say and what we do or, to put it another way, the gap between what we espouse and the lived experience. We all do this and of course we all want to paint a better image of ourselves than what we (subconsciously) know to be the reality.

Paying attention to language provides a window into these contradictions, incongruities and blind spots. So, to gauge where you and your key stakeholders are in terms of understanding of person-centredness, a 'language exercise' is a useful activity. Doing this exercise with individuals or in groups creates a focus for discussion and dialogue about different perspectives on person-centredness and different understandings of the words we use to talk about it. It also starts the process of thinking about a vision and the values that might be important to pay attention to as we develop the curriculum.

Here are two methods of undertaking a language exercise that you might find useful. These methods were developed in a large strategic programme in the Irish Health Service (McCormack et al. 2022).

Our Language! How Person Centred are We?

INFORMATION FOR PERSONS USING AND PROVIDING A SERVICE

As part of a process of changing our culture to a more person-centred culture, we are going to look at the language we use in our everyday practice to see how person centred or non-person centred it is. This exercise involves everyone as we all contribute to the language used and to the culture we experience as staff as well as persons using services and their families.

WHAT WILL HAPPEN?

A language exercise will take place over a few weeks, and you are invited to take part. This exercise is for everyone, and we ask that you contribute freely and as often as you wish over this time. We would like you to think about the language you use and hear used every day and start to question whether you think it is person centred or not. There are several ways we can do this, and we will share this with you so that you know how to become involved.

When the exercise is finished, we will look at what has come up and agree together, what language we have said is no longer acceptable for us to use and what we want to replace it with. This is not an exercise in political correctness as that is about what's in fashion. This is about using language that shows respect for the person as a unique individual – persons using and providing services. Please embrace this as a learning exercise that you can have fun with as well as learn from. It is about the language we use to talk and write about each other and this includes colleagues as well as persons using services and their families. Look at what we say, how we write and our signage.

There are different ways of approaching this exercise. You could use flipcharts headed as below put in prominent places where everyone can see, along with an invitation to everyone to take part (CIP).

There are a few examples below to start you off but there are lots more.

Non- or less person-centred language used	Suggest more person-centred language
My team	Our team
The managers/staff/girls/lads	Colleagues
Dear all (on emails)	Hello (name of person) or everybody
Homework	Precourse reading
The kids	Learners
Pet names, e.g. love, pet, etc. Patronising terms, e.g. 'you are so good'	Person's name Thank you!

You might like to consider using a 'language tree' where words can be written on different coloured leaves that represent person-centred and non-person-centred language used. This can be a real tree/branches or made. Use CIP principles of collaboration, inclusion and participation to figure out what method you want to use.

QUESTIONS YOU MIGHT ASK YOURSELF WHEN THINKING ABOUT THIS EXERCISE

- Why does it matter if my language is person centred or not?
- How do I contribute to person-centredness through my language?
- How can I make my language more person centred?
- How can I make a difference?
- What do we do next?

CHANGE TAKES TIME

Changing language takes time as often words and phrases have been in use for a long time. So please be patient with each other and us but also please stick with it too. We will agree how we can all supportively challenge each other when we slip up, probably doing this in a fun way.

We will plan together how we will evaluate our language on a regular basis to see if we are getting there and we would welcome all ideas as to how we can do this.

Have fun!

Facilitating a Language Exercise in Groups

Purpose: to raise awareness of language used that is and is not person centred
Intended outcome: (i) more person-centred language used that represents shared values and beliefs about person-centredness; (ii) a means of evaluating workplace culture
Process: language exercise
Time: 1 hour 30 minutes

CONTEXT

Most of us are unaware of the everyday language that we use in work. We all adopt phrases and words that are commonly used within the workplace as a way of quickly communicating between each other. Some of these words and phrases are common to all workplaces and others unique to particular settings such as older persons' services, ID services, mental health or acute settings. We become so accustomed

(continued)

(continued)

to using particular words and phrases that we no longer notice them as they have become routine. We also use signage that is very unfriendly: 'keep out', 'staff only', 'no access'. However, language can give away a lot about our collective values and beliefs without us knowing it. Although we may no longer notice this language, people who use services or are new to working in a service will notice. This can become a problem when there are several potential meanings to words or phrases commonly used. What is acceptable to one person may have a completely different meaning to someone else. Although the intention may not be to show disrespect, it is how it can be felt by the other person that is important.

The only way we can really understand the impact of our language is to critically look at the everyday phrases we use and hear used, spoken or written, and question whether or not they show respect for the person as an individual. In order to raise awareness within the culture change group, you need to provide active learning space to explore together words that could have the potential to convey a submessage of disrespect, however unintentional.

ACTIVITY

1. Using a flipchart, choose a word or phrase in common use within the group and write it in large print in the centre of the page. This word could be 'the girls', 'the elderly', 'my team', 'the feeds', 'dear all' 'the management', etc.
2. Ask everyone to call out as many words as they can that they associate with this word or phrase without overthinking it. Make sure you contribute also if you are part of that culture or service.
3. Write all contributions around the word/phrase in the middle of the page and make sure you do not rate any contributions or open any conversation at this stage on a particular word.
4. Keep it going until you have filled the page or you come to a natural stop.
5. Together, look at what is on the page and ask what people are seeing. At this stage, it usually occurs to people that there are a lot of words that have different meanings or associations. Some are positive but many can be negative. Have a dialogue about the difference between person-centred words that respect the individuality of us all versus words that are fashionable that are not necessarily person centred, for example 'millennial', 'silver surfers', etc. Discuss the use of pet names rather than the person's preferred name: 'love', 'dear'. Remember it is not about your intention – it is how it can make the other person feel when they are not called by their name. Did anyone ever say 'Call me love' instead of their name? Asking people if they mind does not work – why? Because there is usually a power imbalance between staff and between staff and persons using the service. A good example is 'the girls or lads', rarely used between senior people who refer to each other by name in general but could refer to those less senior to them. This open conversation helps everyone, including you, learn from each other.

6. Divide a flipchart page in half and put the headings 'Person-centred language I use/hear used' and on the other side 'Language I think is not person centred that I use/hear used'. If it is a big group, divide in half, but if small stay together and make sure you take part. Have a dialogue about what has come up.
7. The next stage is planning how to bring this back to the workplace.

EXPLORING CULTURE AND CONTEXT – HOW TO DEVELOP PERSON-CENTRED LEARNING CULTURES

Much of what you learn in this book will be about developing person-centred learning cultures. Everything we do and how we interact and connect with others shape the culture through direction, action and influence. In this section, we are going to start at the foundation of culture and consider the place of values and beliefs in strategy. By setting out the values and beliefs that underpin the curriculum strategy, an organisation is making explicit the espoused values underpinning ways of being, doing and becoming that are important to developing person-centred healthcare practitioners – the mission of any healthcare curriculum.

Manley et al. (2011) set out a framework for effective workplace culture that identifies the characteristics of such a culture. We have adapted this framework, drawing on our learning from developing the person-centred curriculum framework and other strategic work in person-centred culture change.

Attributes of a Person-centred Context

1. Specific values shared and realised in the setting where learning takes place, namely:
   - commitment to person-centred lifelong learning
   - high support and high challenge
   - leadership development
   - involvement, collaboration and participation by stakeholders
   - evidence use and development
   - positive attitude to change
   - open communication
   - teamwork
   - safety (holistic).
2. There is a shared vision and mission and individual and collective responsibility for working towards achieving them.
3. Adaptability, innovation and creativity for learning effectiveness.
4. Appropriate change is driven by the needs of communities of learners.
5. Formal systems (structures and processes) enable continuous evaluation of learning and performance.

(continued)

(continued)

FACTORS THAT ENABLE THE CONTEXT TO BE REALISED

Individual factors

- Person-centred leadership
- Skilled facilitation
- Clarity of role

Organisational factors

- An enabling approach to management, leadership and decision making
- Organisational readiness
- Person-centred approaches to people and performance management

EXPECTED OUTCOMES

Evidence that:

(a) the needs of communities of learners are met in a person-centred way
(b) staff are empowered and committed
(c) standards, goals and objectives are met (individual, team and organisational effectiveness)
(d) knowledge/evidence is developed, used and shared
(e) healthful cultures are developed
(f) human flourishing for all is encouraged.

Considering these characteristics in the shaping of a strategy is important as they form a basis for identifying domains of practice that need to be included when developing an effective learning culture.

DEVELOPING SHARED VALUES, VISION AND MISSION

Identifying Values at a Strategic Level

Identifying values at a strategic level is about planning for success and this means having conversations about values and cultures in organisations. Simply put, values are important to stakeholders connected with the organisation, either directly as employees or indirectly as collaborators, partners, etc. It is vital to spend time clarifying these values as some stakeholders may not know what the espoused organisational values are, while others may have differing views of the values that are important. At the strategic level, values express what is core to the organisation. Strategic values can be clarified and refined as part of the process of co-developing the vision and mission of the organisation. The mission statement is about purpose and the desired end-goal, whereas strategy is about making explicit the strategic goals and associated actions necessary to realise the vision.

Chapter 5 focuses specifically on 'shared values' in a curriculum. In that chapter, translation of the person-centred strategy into learning cultures that enable the curriculum to be operationalised will be explored. If you wish to engage in a process with strategic stakeholders to develop shared values for the curriculum, then please go to Chapter 5 where you will find a variety of tools and processes that can be used for this purpose.

Developing a Mission Statement and Shared Vision

In setting out a strategic roadmap, it is prudent to develop a mission statement and a shared vision. A mission statement makes explicit the strategic purpose, reason for being and core values. Mission statements are often formed as a corporate indication of an organisation's remit. Aligned with a mission statement, a team may also agree a shared vision. The shared vision additionally communicates the intentions of the team, capturing the positive impact that the team collectively aspires to achieve, including goals or objectives that may be time-oriented (e.g. short, medium or long term).

A critical element of developing a mission statement and shared vision is that they are co-created through participative, inclusive and collaborative endeavour. Without a foundation of shared values and a process of co-creation, there is a risk that both may lack authenticity and ownership, rendering them redundant. However, the positive counterclaim holds greater appeal. Where the mission statement emanates from the team, with an authentic commitment to an agreed value proposition and a strategy to realise it, an impetus for transformation can be ignited via which desired prospects become reality. When aligned with shared values, the mission statement and shared vision acknowledge what people believe, think and feel is important, thereby engaging minds and hearts to identify what team members value and are willing to commit to progressing together.

In the context of person-centredness in healthcare curricula, the mission statement and shared vision will focus on the value proposition which is the unique selling point for stakeholders. The mission statement and shared vision will reflect that learning about person-centred practice is of strategic, educational, legal, professional and clinical significance, and offer a shared aspiration of what person-centredness in healthcare curricula can achieve for individuals, teams and persons in need of healthcare.

The greater the involvement of all key stakeholders in creating the mission statement, the more inspirational the potential for transformative change. It therefore follows that the processes used to create the mission statement are crucial to its realisation. A strong bond and sense of purpose are created when stakeholders share a common vision that has been created together, rather than one they have been given. Most stakeholders, like most people, want to be a part of something bigger, and a mission statement that communicates a shared vision provides this by making aspirations intentional. The mission statement establishes the agreed direction of travel and a focus on which to channel contributions, energy and innovation. Without a mission statement, stakeholders may feel a lack of direction and disenchantment, where the pursuit of individual interests may be tangential to espoused values and the stakeholders' collective purpose and progress.

As well as providing focus, coherence and direction, a mission statement and shared vision constitute a baseline platform from which to evaluate current practices and the learning culture. This will help you to make decisions about how suggested new ways of working will contribute to movement towards achieving the shared vision. The mission statement and shared vision can therefore be used as a point of reference on which to focus, guide and refocus the intentions of everyday practices.

Shared visions emerge from personal visions that emanate from values and beliefs. Expression of personal values and beliefs is thus central to successfully contributing to a collaborative vision within your team. Depending on the team and people you are working with, and the time you have for this work, you may need to do some preparatory work to help people to talk about their personal visions (based on their own values and beliefs). However, it is possible to undertake values and beliefs work and then move straight into shared vision work all together.

Weaving in elements of the background information offered above on developing a mission statement and shared vision, as you introduce and facilitate vision work, may assist groups to make more sense of the purpose of developing a shared vision. Where people in the team have different cultural experiences, language skills and ways of understanding, you might need to explain what a shared vision is in words and ways they can understand. This may, for example, include images that portray key principles.

In the next section of this chapter, we have set out various workshop activities for developing a mission statement and shared vision. We encourage you to use the methods as set out here before you try to amend them. This is just so you can be confident and competent in delivering the core stages of the method before adding your own touches or becoming more adventurous.

Using Creativity

Introducing creativity helps to balance left brain activity (rational, analytical thinking) with right brain activity (creative imagination) and is more likely to release greater potential and achieve a fuller range of options. Bringing in creative methods helps us to use our imaginations and creativity to build a vision for person-centredness in healthcare curricula. They can also be more fun!

Some team members may have creative hobbies and use creative arts but for many, working with creativity, especially in the workplace, is a new experience. We have found that people experience a variety of feelings in response to the prospect of exploring the use of their creative imagination. These feelings may include shyness, embarrassment, anxiety, excitement and pleasure. These are all natural and usual responses to new ways of learning and engaging in learning. It is vital that a facilitator creates a safe and open space in which everyone who takes part can explore and learn in new ways.

You may find it useful to encourage people to reflect on how they feel about participating in a workshop with creative methods, and to think about the kinds of support strategies they would find helpful. In our experience, feedback on creative methods included comments such as 'sceptical and then sold', 'felt a bit vulnerable/self-conscious, but see its potential value', 'very good, more of this type of work would be useful', 'amazed at its power', 'great opportunity to see and experience visioning'.

How To Do It: Creative Methods for Developing a Shared Vision: Programme of Three Workshops (You Decide Which One You Might Do)

These workshops provide opportunities for new facilitators to work in person-centred ways with small groups. The workshops link with the values clarification method exercise. Participants will build on the work they have done to clarify their own values and beliefs and use it to build a vision together. Participants will practise a key skill of being person centred – the capacity to accept that others may have different values, experiences and views to theirs. They will be able to practise listening attentively to others and not being judgemental or trying to interpret the other people's expressions of their visions.

VISUALISATION THROUGH PAINTING AND/OR COLLAGE

In this 1.5-hour workshop, people will be invited to create a painting or collage that reflects their vision and aspirations of their education practice and workplace. It is based on the idea that creating something helps us to understand what the future might look like, and it can also help us to start talk about what needs to happen to make the vision real. There will be a conversation about what emerges. You will have the opportunity to practise using creativity as a means of bringing up values that are so much a part of us that they are difficult to talk about.

VISIONING

This creative workshop is shorter and can be done in 30–45 minutes, so if time is tight, then you may choose this option. Through creative visualisation, the facilitator takes people on an imaginary journey through which they explore whatever comes spontaneously into their imagination, using all the senses (imaginatively). You will have the chance to stretch your mind and open up to new ways of doing things.

VISION STATEMENT DEVELOPMENT

While vision work is always going to involve an element of imagination about what might and could be, some people may find it difficult to engage in the creative approaches above. Thus, this one-hour workshop may be more suitable for people who prefer to work through analysis and discussion. In this workshop, a vision statement can be generated from the summary of the values clarification exercise. You will be able to practise involving everyone in reaching agreement.

How To Do It – Workshop Guidance: Visualisation Through Painting and/or Collage

This group activity would give a new facilitator a chance to practise helping people in a small group (maximum of eight) to work together effectively. If possible, the new facilitator could also work alongside a more experienced facilitator for a group of 20–25.

AIM

The aim of this workshop is for team members to develop a shared personal vision for the future that will guide the practice development work. Depending on your service, you may also want to include other partners and stakeholders.

ACTIVITIES

People will be invited to create a painting or collage that reflects their vision and aspirations of their practice and workplace. Creating something generates understanding about what the future is going to look like and people can begin to open up, talking about what needs to happen to make the vision real.

RESOURCES

- 1.5 hours.
- A large room with chairs around the side and some tables for those who want to work on a surface.
- One or two facilitators (usually two facilitators for 20–25 participants).
- Materials for painting; felt-tip pens, crayons, pastels (plus any other drawing materials you want to include); newspaper or other floor covering if paint is being used.
- Materials for collage include the above plus magazines and newspapers or a supply of images; clay, scissors, glue sticks; everyday small leftover and 'junk' items (e.g. wine bottle tops/corks, plastic containers), leaves, flowers, small twigs and branches, silver-coloured foil, coloured paper, tissue papers and card, felt.
- A flipchart easel, paper and marker pens.

FORMAT

Introduction and purpose of workshop (5 minutes).

Creative work individually in a quiet or silent space (15 minutes).

Ask participants to organise themselves into small groups where each individual shares the meaning of their painting or collage and the group records on flipchart sheets the key attributes of each personal vision (15 minutes).

Open gallery viewing and sharing of paintings and collages and the creator's intended message (15 minutes).

If you have longer and want to include a discussion at this point, you can achieve this by inviting responses on the work based on the following:

- I see...
- I feel...
- I imagine...

Do not encourage discussion about the 'artistic' quality of the work or viewers telling the creator of the work what the work means.

Discussion in the large group or several smaller groups based on the key questions (45 minutes).

- What is our shared vision for future practice?
- What are the key features of future practice?
- How will we move towards our new vision?

Summarise the purpose of the work and the emerging points and suggest that participants consider what they have learned from the creative method. Outline what will happen next to build on the collaborative work.

How To Do It – Workshop Guidance: Creating and Sharing Personal Visions

This workshop can be offered to team members and other stakeholders by an experienced facilitator. If possible, a novice facilitator could experience the visualisation as a participant and then work alongside the experienced facilitator by writing on the flipchart, for example.

AIM

To share and develop a mission statement with stakeholders in a healthcare education setting.

RESOURCES

Time: 30–45 minutes.

(continued)

(continued)

ACTIVITIES

First create a space in the room, pushing back tables and chairs if necessary. Invite people to make themselves comfortable, on a chair or on the floor. You might like to put something in the centre, on the floor, for example a jug of flowers or leaves and a candle and play some gentle music. The space is now ready for the visioning exercise.

Explain that the purpose of this session is to help people to use their creative imagination to create their own personal vision for person-centredness in the curriculum in the future. Visioning in this way helps us to tap into areas that are usually difficult to talk about, either because there are no words for it or because it is so deeply ingrained in us that we take it for granted and do not normally talk about it.

The overall method is to take people on a journey in which they explore whatever comes into their imagination, using all the senses (imaginatively). It is important not to get in the way of people's imagination, so the facilitator might say something like this:

> We will be imagining with all our senses, where we have been (in relation to the learning we support and people we have worked with and learned from), where we would like healthcare curricula to go and how we could get there. It is really important on this journey that you participate in a way that feels right for you. Please do not push yourself to follow my suggestions if they do not feel right. Do your own thing. Also, try to go with whatever comes into your imagination, however bizarre, and do not try to analyse it away. Our imagination often holds just the right message for us.

Begin with an exercise that helps people to become grounded. This often involves closing our eyes (except the facilitator) and becoming aware of our own breathing. For example:

> I suggest that we start with a grounding exercise, which will help us to let go of our busyness or whatever we have been doing and come into the 'here and now' and be truly present. Close your eyes now and listen to the sounds outside the room. We are going to leave the outside world for a time, letting go, for now, our thoughts about all our responsibilities at work and at home and our hopes, fears and expectations for this visioning session. Bring your attention to the sounds inside this room (pause). And now, to the sounds within yourself. Listen to your breath (pause) and feeling the rise and fall of the chest (pause). Letting go as we breathe out (pause).

Then help people into an imaginary scene, for example a country landscape, beside the sea, up in the sky, a city dwelling – whatever, using any of a number of devices, such as going down through the earth by following the roots of a tree or going up to the sky by following the branches or walking across different kinds of ground. Invite people to choose a way in that is right and feels safe for them (say, for example,

'If you do not want to go through the earth, you might like to set out on an imaginary walk across a muddy field, along a beach or in a city'). Thus, we are sensitive to those who might feel fears such as claustrophobia or who have a fear of heights. Encourage people to accept the scene that opens up before them.

Explore the past, future and present by going to the place that represents what it was like to learn and/or teach in the past, the future and the present. Invite participants to journey back to that past. When they get there, suggest they move, in their imagination, around their past. Ask them the following.

What do you:

- see?
- hear?
- taste?
- smell?
- feel (touch and emotions)?

After what feels like an appropriate amount of quiet or silence, invite participants to start moving towards their future in supporting learning in any way that springs from their imagination. Suggest they notice what they see, hear, smell, taste and feel on this part of the journey. When they arrive at their future, ask participants to really focus on noticing as much as they can and taking notice of their emotions. After a while, suggest they look back over their shoulder at where they have come from in their past. After a period of quiet or silence, invite participants to set off back to the present and the curricula, teaching and learning today and then to explore it and imagine how they would get from this to the person-centred approach of the future.

Bring people back to the actual present, into the room, by retracing their steps, for example helping them come back through the earth or along the branches back to the base of the tree or whatever. Give people time. When they emerge, you might say:

When you are ready, gently open your eyes. If you would like to, pair up for a few minutes with someone near you and share your experience of past, future, present and how you made the journey from present to future. Or, you may prefer to spend the time alone and make a few notes or a drawing of what you have experienced.

Then invite sharing in the larger group about what they imagined and/or about the experience of visioning. The facilitator then asks participants to think about their experience and how this can be related to the way the team currently works with people. This part of the work can be carried out through small group discussion and using flipchart recordings to capture the vision statement and its features and how it is different from what happens now.

(continued)

(continued)

While some participants report that they get a lot out of this method, others say it does very little or even nothing for them. So, you will need to have a repertoire of methods for visioning and to know when the time is right to bring in any of the creative imagination methods. At the same time, gentle encouragement of participants to use their creative imagination in visioning work offers new learning experiences for stretching the mind and trying something new. It's vital to bring the imaginative element back to what this means for your care setting and the way care is organised and delivered.

How To Do It – Workshop Guidance: Vision Statement Development

The workshop should be facilitated by someone who has experienced the values clarification exercise as some of the processes are similar.

AIM

The aim of this method is to generate a shared vision statement about person-centredness in your healthcare curriculum that sets out the aspirations of the team. The processes of the workshop itself will help you to learn how to be democratic and person centred in the ways you work together. In other words, that everyone has a voice in creating and agreeing the shared vision statement.

CONTEXT

Vision work involves an element of imagination about what might and can be. Thus, the creative methods enable creativity to come to the fore. If this is felt to be inappropriate for any reason, a vision statement can be generated from the summary of the values and beliefs work.

WHAT IS A SHARED VISION STATEMENT?

A vision statement comprises a summary of:

- the ultimate purpose of .... (e.g. our work in supporting learning and the development of person-centred practice)
- how that purpose can best be achieved
- what factors will help with the achievement of the shared vision.

RESOURCES

- One hour.
- A large room with chairs well spaced out.
- One or two facilitators (usually two facilitators to 20–25 participants).
- Flipchart easel, paper and marker pens.
- Flipchart sheets with the sticky notes that captured the themes from the values clarification exercise and the draft summary statements from that exercise.

ACTIVITIES

The participants are divided into three groups and the facilitator provides cues and instructions for the activity.

Each group takes one of the draft summary statements from the values clarification work and ensures that there is a coherent summary statement written that captures the themes generated from the values clarification exercise (15 minutes).

The groups identify any jargon or confusing terminology in the statement and debate the possible meanings of the terms until agreement is reached (20 minutes).

Each group then shares the terminology that was under debate and the proposed agreed meanings. The other groups have an opportunity to question or add further debate until agreement is reached. The facilitators' focus is to promote open discussion and guide the groups to reach agreement (20 minutes).

Summary statements may need to be rewritten depending on the outcome of the group work. Any key points needed or clarification of terms are captured on flipchart sheets. The facilitator summarises the session, or asks the participants to summarise the session, and identify individual learning and its relationship to developing educational practice. Action points for the next steps can be negotiated. The key aspects of this session are to promote an active debate on taken-for-granted jargon or confusing terns to ensure that the group has a shared understanding of meaning. This helps with clarity in the vision work and also enables participants to be more consistent when talking with others about the vision.

ACTIVITY 2.2

How Will We Embody and Enact Our Shared Vision?

Once a shared vision has been created and agreed, it is important that you facilitate a discussion about the team's expectations of what needs to happen to ensure the vision becomes reality. You might use questions such as the following.

- How will we help each other to work to achieve our shared vision?
- How will we make use of this mission statement in our everyday practice to support learning?

TRANSLATING THE STRATEGIC VISION INTO PRACTICE

In this chapter, we have considered how stakeholders could develop healthful learning cultures through values clarification and forming a mission statement and shared vision. In the next chapters, we will examine how teams could translate these strategic intentions into the workings of the curriculum. We will explore the structures, systems, leadership styles, staff knowledge and skills needed for this work to happen. As already stated, Chapter 5 specifically focuses on shared values and how to make these real in practice.

Engaging Authentically and Meaningfully

There has been an increasing focus in quality improvement, research and policy development of engagement with key stakeholders to achieve optimal outcomes. This requires everyone's commitment in all stages of the process to promote learning and achieve desired outcomes.

Engaging authentically is a prerequisite to developing and realising a shared vision. This pivots on developing positive interactive relationships, identifying aims, process and collaboration to achieve the intended outcomes. Centrally, this translates to working with our own and other people's values in a safe space underpinned by mutual respect. Bringing people together is the first step and we provide some activities that can help clarify shared values and beliefs so that a shared vision can be agreed on what direction to take and to foster empowerment of the group towards the collective vision.

A central aim is to create a reality where people own the vision as it is personally relevant for them and where personal visions are integrated to shared vision. We show you activities to open these conversations and work towards an agreed shared vision.

Authentic collaboration means explicitly championing a no-blame environment and that everyone's voice matters and every perspective is important. From this stance, we can determine what we want and what we need to do to make that a successful reality.

Identifying and Engaging Stakeholders

There will be a diverse range of people, groups and organisations who will be affected by, or have an interest in, the development and delivery of a person-centred curriculum and are therefore potential stakeholders. It is likely that people will want to be included and participate in varying degrees and ways and at different times. There will also be people who have a bigger part to play and who we consider key stakeholders.

There are many tools and approaches available in the literature that enable a considered and strategic approach to the identification of key stakeholders. Irrespective of the approach you choose, the following are some key questions to be considered.

- Who will you need to work with directly?
- Who has decision-making power?
- Who has the resources that may be required?
- Who has the skills that may be required?
- Who will actively support or promote the process?

An activity to enable you to begin this process is described below.

ACTIVITY 2.3

Identifying Key Stakeholders

You can do this activity within your immediate team, with someone taking the lead to structure the activities. You will need:

- 20–30 minutes
- a copy of this sheet of instructions
- a flipchart and pens.

On the flipchart sheet, write the names of everyone the group thinks are key stakeholders. Help them to think widely as there are likely to be individuals or services that might not at first come to mind, but who might influence the development of a person-centred curriculum or be affected by it. Such people might turn out to be your biggest support or the biggest resisters to change. Stick this flipchart sheet on the wall if possible.

- Now draw three circles – one inside the other – on a new sheet.
- Identify who in the list are your key stakeholders that you need to work directly with and write their names in the centre circle.
- In the next circle going out, write the names of those you need to consult.
- And in the next circle, those you need to keep informed.
- Check that you have included everyone on the list in one of the circles.

Once you have identified your key stakeholders, it is useful to undertake some further work to understand their importance and potential influence. It may not always be those you work with directly that will have the greater influence on the development process. Similarly, there are a variety of stakeholder analysis tools in the literature that will support how you plan to communicate with different stakeholder groups. One such resource can be found at www.projectengineer.net/3-types-of-stakeholder-matrix. The developers of this resource offer three kinds of matrices for analysing power relationships that enable a team to understand the stakeholders' potential interaction with the work. We believe that two of them are particularly valuable in curriculum strategy development.

- *Option 1: The Power–Interest Matrix.* In this context, *power* is the ability of the stakeholder to stop or change the project and *interest* is the level of overlap between the stakeholder's and the project's goals.
- *Option 2: Stakeholder Engagement Assessment Matrix.* This method places stakeholders into five categories: unaware (not aware of the project and its potential impacts on them); resistant (aware of the project but not in support of it); neutral (aware of the project but have no opinion regarding their support for it); supportive (supportive of the project and wish it to succeed); and leading (actively engaged in project success and willing to lend assistance to help it succeed).

Undertaking such a stakeholder analysis will inform the development of a communication plan outlining the different kinds of stakeholders to establish how to

BOX 2.1

Developing a Communication Plan with Stakeholders

Stakeholders	How to communicate	Who will communicate
Those you will work with directly (these people might become members of the practice development co-ordinating group)		
Those you will consult		
Those you will inform		

communicate and who will be responsible for ensuring effective engagement. Box 2.1 provides a simple template for developing a communication plan for stakeholders.

PULLING IT TOGETHER

So far in this chapter, we have explored different components of a person-centred approach to developing an underpinning strategy for your curriculum. How much or little of these activities you will engage in depends on the extent of the strategic work your department has undertaken already and the size of the curriculum development project (e.g. a whole new course versus a single unit of study).

We have suggested a development journey that progresses from general principles to specific activities. However, you will need to bring all these elements together into a strategic plan or map that draws out the key areas that need to be considered as you progress through the rest of the curriculum planning process. As we know from our experiences of developing curricula and from what participants in the curriculum framework development project told us, these strategic visions, missions, values and principles often get 'lost' or at best diluted as the work progresses. Below, we suggest a workshop that can be used to 'pull it all together' and identify key areas of activity that need to be given attention in the rest of the curriculum planning process.

Workshop: Pulling It Together

In this workshop, we will focus on identifying priorities or indicators for action derived from the work you have done in unpacking the four strategic themes.

- Developing a person-centred stance.
- Exploring existing culture and context.
- Developing a shared vision and mission.
- Engaging authentically and meaningfully.

An indicator is a key theme that indicates issues or areas that may be worth investigating further or prioritising in your ongoing curriculum development work. The purpose of this workshop is to discuss whether any of these indicators are worth further investigation or attention in the curriculum development plan.

You will need:

- approximately two hours (or 2 × 1-hour sessions)
- copies of the final sets of data, information, feedback, stakeholder analysis, vision statements, etc. that you have collected and developed so far
- a facilitator
- copies of the person-centred practice curriculum framework template (below)
- a flipchart and pens
- a room with tables for small groups of 4–6.

KEY ACTIVITIES

- In advance of the workshop, ideally the final sets of data, information, feedback, stakeholder analysis, vision statements, etc. are typed up and circulated to group members to consider. If this is not possible then handwritten notes will do so long as they are readable by others.

(continued)

(continued)

- Begin by sharing the agreed vision and seeking any final comments and views. Keep the vision visible to all workshop participants so that all discussion connects with it and is focused on moving towards achieving the vision.
- Then invite the small groups to discuss the issues, feedback and data as well as your interpretations of these. For example, they might discuss lack of person-centred competence (feedback): feedback from service directors that current graduates do not seem to have a firm grasp of what it means to be person centred and thus get caught up in the busyness of the work and ignore the person (interpretation).
- Indicators would then be identified for consideration as areas of focus in developing the other parts of the person-centred practice curriculum framework. For example, the category of 'lack of person-centred competence' might be identified as one of the indicators that must have priority attention in the skills part of the framework, with potential indicators being identified, such as being present, getting to know the person, working with a patient's beliefs and values, etc. The indicators are put on a flipchart and presented to the other groups for discussion.
- Help the whole group to reach agreement on the indicators and which have priority. Using the person-centred practice curriculum framework template, invite the small groups to map the agreed indicators (there is a filled-in template below to help you understand what we mean), then to share their mapping with the other groups.
- Help the whole group reach agreement on how an overview plan that takes the prioritised indicators into account could be made and potentially by whom. It is likely that several mini-projects will fall out of the overview plan and each mini-project would develop its own curriculum development plan with reference to the overview plan.
- Agree how the findings can be fed back to stakeholders to comment on before proceeding with developing the plan.

Person-centred Practice Curriculum Framework Template

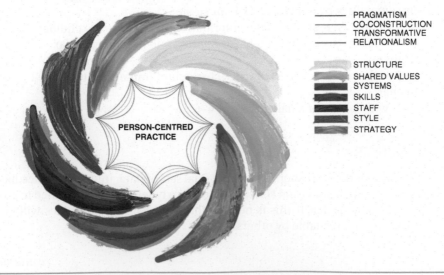

——— PRAGMATISM
——— CO-CONSTRUCTION
——— TRANSFORMATIVE
——— RELATIONALISM

STRUCTURE
SHARED VALUES
SYSTEMS
SKILLS
STAFF
STYLE
STRATEGY

PERSON-CENTRED PRACTICE

Strategic issues identified as indicators	Shared values	Structure	Systems	Skills	Staff	Style
Lack of person-centred competence	Getting to know the person			Being present. Working with a person's beliefs and values		

SUMMARY

In this chapter, we have begun the curriculum development process with a focus on 'strategy' as the foundation for the rest of the work you will undertake as you progress through the process. As you will have seen from this chapter, we are encouraging a collaborative, inclusive and participative approach to doing this work embedded in the same person-centred values and practices that we want to see as outcomes of learning for those participating in a programme. Developing person-centred ways of being and doing is not a one-off module, unit or short course. Instead, learners need to see the values and practices lived out through all stages of the curriculum development, implementation and evaluation. The outcomes arising from the work undertaken to develop this strategy will inform how you engage in the ongoing development processes, ways of working that you can try out and a commitment to meaningful engagement with all stakeholders.

REFERENCES

Carvalho, M., Cabral, I., Verdasca, J.L., and Alves, J.M. (2021). Strategy and strategic leadership in education: a scoping review. *Frontiers in Education* 6: 706608.

Dickson, C., van Lieshout, F., Kmetec, S. et al. (2020). Developing philosophical and pedagogical principles for a pan-European person-centred curriculum framework. *International Practice Development Journal* 10 (2): (Special Issue).

Gruden, M.K., Turk, E., McCormack, B., and Stiglic, G. (2020). Impact of person-centered interventions on patient outcomes in acute care settings – a systematic review. *Journal of Nursing Care Quality* 36 (1): E14–E21.

Haas, M. and Mortensen, M. (2016). The secrets of great teamwork. *Harvard Business Review* 94 (6): 70–76.

Health Foundation (2016). Person-centred Care Made Simple. What Everyone Should Know About Person-centred Care. www.health.org.uk/sites/default/files/PersonCentr.edCare-MadeSimple.pdf.

Lorde, A. (1977). The Transformation of Silence into Language and Action. www.buriedinprint.com/audre-lordes-the-transformation-of-silence-into-language-and-action-1977.

Manley, K., Sanders, K., Cardiff, S., and Webster, J. (2011). Effective workplace culture: the attributes, enabling factors and consequences of a new concept. *International Practice Development Journal* 1 (2): 1–29.

McCormack, B. (2022). Person-centred care and measurement: the more one sees, the better one knows where to look. *Journal of Health Services Research and Policy.* 27 (2): 85–87.

McCormack, B. and McCance, T. (2017). *Person-Centred Nursing and Health Care – Theory and Practice.* Oxford.: Wiley.

McCormack, B., Baldie, D., Peelo-Kilroe, L., and Codd, M. (2022). The HSE National Facilitator Development Programme: Enabling Cultures of Person-Centredness. www.hse.ie/eng/about/who/nqpsd/qps-education/person-centred-programme.html.

Odeh, G. (2021). Implementing McKinsey 7S model of organizational diagnosis and planned change, best Western Italy case analysis. *Journal of International Business and Management* 11 (4): 1–8.

Peters, T.J. and Waterman, R.H. (1982). *In Search of Excellence: Lessons from America's Best-Run Companies.* New York: Harper & Row.

Rotthoff, T., Kadmon, M., and Harendza, S. (2021). It does not have to be either or! Assessing competence in medicine should be a continuum between an analytic and a holistic approach. *Advances in Health Sciences Education* 26 (5): 1659–1673.

Van Schalkwyk, S.C., Hafler, J., Brewer, T.F. et al. for the Bellagio Global Health Education Initiative(2019). Transformative learning as pedagogy for the health professions: a scoping review. *Medical Education* 53 (6): 547–558.

Waterman, R. Jr., Peters, T., and Phillips, J.R. (1980). Structure is not organisation. *Business Horizons* 23 (3): 14–26.

World Health Organization (2007). *People-centred Healthcare: A Policy Framework.* Geneva: WHO.

CHAPTER 3

Structure

In this chapter, we begin by exploring what is meant by the structure of a person-centred curriculum. We consider how curriculum structure fosters learning about person-centredness and creates the conditions for transformative learning and practice. To do this, we invite you to challenge yourself to imagine both what is possible and how these possibilities can be realised through curricular structures. We will also consider how structure helps to establish stakeholder groups that foster curriculum co-design and implementation and explore the structures needed for learners and other stakeholders to participate fully in person-centred curriculum development. Finally, we consider the dynamics of curricular structures and explore how evaluation can inform curriculum validation and renewal, assuring the currency of and fitness for purpose of a curriculum in preparing students for contemporary practice. As in other chapters, throughout this one, we offer a range of activities that will enable you to explore the structure of your own curriculum and how it contributes to the development of person-centred healthcare practitioners.

INTRODUCTION

In this chapter we focus on the 'structure' component of the Person-centred Curriculum Framework. Person-centred curricula are constructivist, increasing in complexity as learners move through programmes. Constructivist theory contends that learning is an active process whereby knowledge is continuously assimilated in response to our experiences of the world. Aligned with this approach, person-centred curricula offer learners flexibility in what is learned, as well as when and how to learn. Key stakeholders are involved in the co-design of the curriculum and its delivery, and robust, ongoing evaluation processes that facilitate collaborative learning for continuous quality improvement are employed. By viewing a 'curriculum' as an open system, rather than confining our view of modules/units/courses as structure to achieve the curriculum

Developing Person-Centred Cultures in Healthcare Education and Practice: An Essential Guide, First Edition.
Edited by Brendan McCormack.
© 2024 John Wiley & Sons Ltd. Published 2024 by John Wiley & Sons Ltd.

intentions, we give attention to the structure of the organisation or department where the learning happens. By focusing on 'structure', we consider learner/stakeholder engagement processes that we embed across the learning organisation, to meet the intended regulatory requirements and ensure that the learning experience meets quality standards.

As the Person-centred Curriculum Framework is synergistic with the Person-centred Practice Framework, the idea of personhood remains at its heart (McCance and McCormack 2021). The intention of all person-centred practices, be they clinical practice, leadership or education, is a healthful culture (see Chapter 2), so learners must experience person-centredness if they are to be person centred. The curriculum structure must therefore support such a culture.

We will begin by outlining the philosophical principles that underpin the Person-centred Curriculum Framework.

Philosophical Principles Underpinning Curriculum Structure

In the early stages of this project previously identified in Chapter 1, Dickson et al. (2020) evaluated stakeholders' views of person-centred curricula across Europe with the aim of identifying key philosophical principles commensurate with person-centredness in healthcare curricula. The philosophical principles (transformative, co-constructed, relational and pragmatic) highlight core considerations when designing a curriculum with person-centredness at its heart. They are the cornerstones of the Person-centred Curriculum Framework and the reference point for any discussion about curricular structures. A brief introduction to each principle is provided as a basis for further reference and reflection.

A Person-centred Curriculum is Transformative

This principle is concerned with how person-centred curricula harness the potential for transformative learning and practice. This can be achieved by challenging individuals to examine their ways of being and doing, by expanding their consciousness and developing new perspectives that stimulate positive action. The transformative potential is relevant to all those who engage in learning. Curricula that are transformative facilitate learners and educators to develop the self-knowledge, confidence and competence needed to be self-regulating, empathetic and collaborative healthcare professionals.

A Person-centred Curriculum is Co-constructed

A curriculum that is co-constructed acknowledges the fundamental premise that person-centred approaches to learning and practice value personhood and collaborative ways of working. Mutual respect is a key principle of both co-design and person-centred practice, and thus all views and contributions are equally valued in the curricular engagement processes. Being inclusive, participative, respectful, iterative and outcome focused are key indicators of mutual respect in co-design (Brand et al. 2021). Inclusivity means that all those who have a stake in the curriculum (i.e. learners, healthcare consumers, healthcare professionals, educators, commissioners) have the opportunity and support to be included in all stages of the curriculum development process. Curriculum co-design is viewed as an iterative process that takes time for all key stakeholders to develop a shared vison of the curriculum. The shared outcome is the achievement of a co-created curriculum that meets the requirements of regulatory systems and organisations as well as being more likely to meet the expressed needs of key stakeholders (Brand et al. 2021).

A Person-centred Curriculum is Relational

In keeping with the values underpinning the concept of personhood, being authentic and demonstrating mutual respect are key components of being person centred and doing person-centred practice. The curriculum therefore needs to be structured in such a way that encourages learners and educators to learn about and know self, as outlined in Chapter 5. It needs to create spaces for connecting with other persons to engage in dialogue and debate in classrooms, in departments and across organisations. Curricular structure considers spaces for voices to be heard and relationships established and nurtured. Relationships between educators and learners, and, educators and educators, are fundamental to achieving successful outcomes and they are made possible by creating psychologically and emotionally safe spaces that foster engagement and shared decision making (see Chapter 4).

A Person-centred Curriculum is Pragmatic

A pragmatic approach to curriculum design affords optimal flexibility in terms of what, when and how learning is organised. This approach is aligned with the principles of autonomy and self-determination, which are indicative of person-centredness. Being pragmatic in curricular structures focuses on seeking new opportunities to be creative in organisational or departmental structures to recognise and respond to students' priorities and learning needs. Pragmatism is also concerned with grounding learner experiences in the real world of practice by embedding scenarios that reflect human experience and context. Examples may include case studies, opportunities for experiential learning and portfolios of assessment.

Chapter 1 explained how the four philosophical principles were applied in the development of the Person-centred Curriculum Framework. The set of thematic actions that were identified arising from the 'structure' component of the Person-centred Curriculum Framework offers ideas for teams to consider within their department. Several examples are shown in Table 3.1. These exemplify some key indicators of person-centredness in curricular structures but are not an exhaustive list. You may be able to think of other ways in which curricular structures are aligned with a person-centred philosophy and educational practices as you work through this chapter. You may also wish to refer to the paper by O'Donnell et al. (2022) for more details about how the thematic actions were derived.

TABLE 3.1   Thematic Actions (Structure).

- Establish an easily accessible, active stakeholder/practice advisory board.
- Map person-centred principles across programmes, in diagrammatic or visual representation to clearly demonstrate links to the curriculum.
- Cultivate personal and professional growth to embody person-centredness with an emphasis on enabling students to use insights as a future professional.
- Foster active learning through negotiated educators/learner autonomy, creativity and flexibility for what is learned and how to enhance intrinsic motivations and learning, balanced against the demands of other stakeholders.
- Inspire learners to take an active role in their education and encourage them to express their feedback, make changes and engage in critical thinking.
- Establish (multi)stakeholder collaborative/communicative spaces, particularly between university and practice contexts and teams, to co-design deliver and evaluate a person-centred curriculum.

FREQUENTLY ASKED QUESTIONS ABOUT STRUCTURE

What is Structure?

Drawing on the philosophical principles, person-centred curricular structures should be authentically co-designed, delivered and evaluated in collaboration with key stakeholders. Structures should also be aligned with the vison of the qualities that are visible in graduates of a specific programme of learning. In a person-centred curriculum, structure therefore refers to how the programme design facilitates and assesses learning in a sequential way, to develop graduates whose practice is person centred. To achieve this, the structure of a person-centred curriculum seeks to introduce and consolidate learning while embedding humanistic values to inform ways of being and doing. We will explore this later in this chapter.

Curriculum structure sets out how learning will be organised, packaged, assessed and developed through each stage of the learning experience so that learners understand and can apply key concepts, enabling them to practise in an effective, accountable and person-centred way (O'Donnell 2021). However, the curriculum structure is a dynamic entity that should also offer learners a degree of flexibility in what is learned, as well as when and how to learn, depending on their learning pace and preferences and within regulatory and programme frameworks.

Where is Structure Visible?

Structures are in operation at multiple levels in educational settings both at organisational and programme levels. For example, at organisational levels, structures may include forums and mechanisms for engagement to facilitate effective communication and business continuity. At programme level, structures provide a frame of reference that direct the sequencing and construction of learning over the duration of a programme. Examples may include programme standards, course documents, module handbooks and practice learning portfolios which collectively provide an overview of the curriculum intentions.

How Would We Know If Our Structure Was Successful?

Structural success depends on establishing and sustaining the physical and organisational approaches needed to construct and sustain the infrastructure of a person-centred curriculum. This includes creating forums with clear terms of reference that facilitate effective engagement and collaborative working with stakeholders, who are aware of and committed to their roles and responsibilities in supporting person-centred learning and practice. Success is also demonstrated through the co-design of curricula that comprehensively and cohesively reflect a person-centred philosophy and principles in the planning and construction of both the theoretical and practical components of the curriculum (O'Donnell 2021).

The overarching indicator of success is the extent to which the curriculum structures provide a robust and contemporary roadmap for the education of learners aligned with the organisational structures to support educators to fully deliver the curriculum as intended.

UNPACKING STRUCTURE THEMES

The thematic actions shown in Table 3.1 help us to think about structures we have in place that enable us to work in person-centred ways, and the spaces, places and timing of engagement with stakeholders. These themes help orientate our attention to how the environment impacts on how we work together, the communication channels we create and how decisions are made. To help us with this, we have structured the rest of this chapter according to four areas of activity.

1. Creating a curriculum structure to develop person-centred educational practice.
2. Creating organisational structures for collaborative, inclusive and participative ways of working that support collective leadership.
3. Creating the conditions for effective partnerships with stakeholders in curriculum design, review and evaluation.
4. Creating spaces to promote learner autonomy so learners can participate fully in person-centred learning.

There are activities within each to help you address person-centred curriculum structure.

Creating A Curriculum Structure to Develop Person-centred Educational Practice

In this section we consider how the architecture of a curriculum is constructed to demonstrate what identifies it as 'person centred'. We will also consider other strategic and operational factors that influence the structure of the curriculum and examine approaches to incorporating these while showcasing the hallmarks of a person-centred curriculum. Activity 3.1 focuses on the requirements and priorities that influence the design of a person-centred curriculum.

ACTIVITY 3.1

Identifying Factors That Influence Curriculum Structure

The purpose of this activity is to identify factors that influence how a curriculum is designed and approved. Gather a core curriculum planning team for a new or existing programme. If there is someone in your organisation who provides guidance on curriculum design, then ask them to join you. To do this activity, you will need two flipchart sheets, sticky notes and pens. Label each of the flipchart chart sheets as shown in Figure 3.1. Stick the flipchart sheets to the wall.

- Individually, and in a quiet space, think of the context in which you support learning. What are the key factors that need to be considered in designing a curriculum? Try to identify both internal and external factors, where external factors relate to influences from outside your institution and internal factors are key considerations in terms of your institution/department/school.
- Record each factor on a sticky note and attach the sticky note to the respective flipchart sheet.
- Discuss the range of influencing factors and identify how you would prioritise these based on factors that are required or optional.

External factors influencing curriculum design	Internal factors influencing curriculum design

FIGURE 3.1 Flipcharts with statements.

In thinking about this activity, you may have identified that for a curriculum or programme to be approved, it needs to satisfy a range of conditions. You may have considered external factors such as accrediting body requirements, professional regulatory or licensing standards, subject benchmarks and workforce priorities. Internal factors may have included perspectives on core disciplinary knowledge, resources (such as technology, staff capabilities, space), cohort size and institutional policies (e.g. regarding assessment practices, etc.). The factors you have identified may be broadly applicable in developing any healthcare curriculum.

In the next activity, we invite you to consider structural features that differentiate a curriculum as person centred.

ACTIVITY 3.2

Identifying the Structural Features of a Person-centred Curriculum

The purpose of this activity is to identify the features of a person-centred curriculum. You should undertake this activity with members of your programme team. You will need a flipchart, pens, sticky dots and sticky notes. Label each of the flipchart sheets as shown in Figure 3.2. Stick the flipchart sheets to the wall.
   Complete each of the following activities.

- Thinking again about the curriculum in which you support learning, each team member is invited to apply a sticky dot to the line shown on flipchart sheet 1, to record the extent to which you each believe the curriculum is person centred.
- What evidence did you consider in making your decision? What we mean is, in what ways is person-centredness explicit in this curriculum and what structures have contributed to its visibility? Record each point on a separate sticky note and add to flipchart sheet 2.
- As a team, discuss what evidence would convince you that person-centredness is fully embedded in a curriculum.

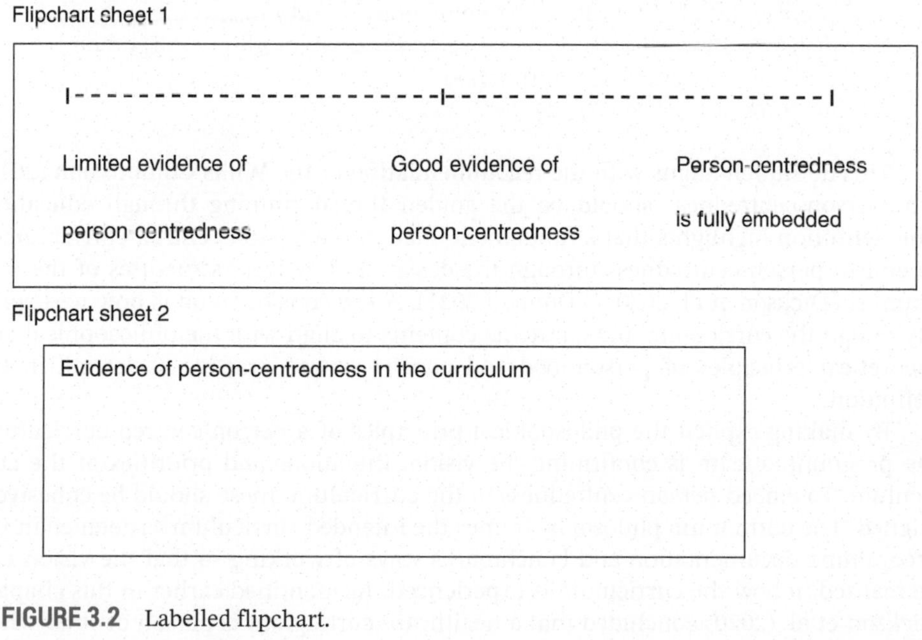

Flipchart sheet 1

| -|- |

| Limited evidence of | Good evidence of | Person-centredness |
| person centredness | person-centredness | is fully embedded |

Flipchart sheet 2

Evidence of person-centredness in the curriculum

FIGURE 3.2   Labelled flipchart.

In undertaking this activity, you may have considered various structural features of a person-centred curriculum. For example, that the curriculum is underpinned by a person-centred philosophy or conceptual framework. You may have concluded that having a module(s)/unit(s) of study that explore aspects of person-centred practice provides evidence of person-centredness in the curriculum. Perhaps your curriculum is person centred as educators facilitate learning and ways of working that are collaborative, offer flexibility and are co-designed with learners. These examples reflect key structural features of a person-centred curriculum. One or more of these hallmarks may be evident in a curriculum. This highlights that person-centredness may be operating at differing levels depending on the structures that are in place.

A useful heuristic may be to consider person-centredness in the curriculum as a continuum rather than an absolute. For example, the programme philosophy may endorse a person-centred approach to healthcare practice that is aligned with the programme content. However, perhaps due to large cohort sizes and the design of learning spaces, teaching, and learning approaches may appear rigid with limited opportunities for person-centred approaches to the facilitation of learning using groupwork or flexibility to respond to learners' needs or priorities. It is important that such tensions are explored and addressed so that the curriculum intentions are lived out in how the curriculum is experienced.

The key hallmark of a person-centred curriculum is in how its structure supports learners to understand and experience person-centredness so that they understand it, recognise it and can apply it to their healthcare practice (O'Donnell et al. 2020). For the purposes of this book, a person-centred curriculum is defined as follows.

> A curriculum is person centred if it is transformative (purpose), grounded in a philosophy of pragmatism (systems world) and enables all learners to co-construct (lifeworld) and experience connectivity with oneself, other persons and contexts (lifeworld) throughout their personal learning journey (see Chapter 1 for further detail).

This definition aligns with the recommendation of the Willis Commission (2012) that person-centredness should be the golden thread running through education. The definition highlights that a fundamental tenet of a person-centred curriculum is to embed person-centredness through the design and delivery structures of the programme (Dickson et al. 2020; O'Donnell 2021). A key consideration is how we explicitly design the curriculum and curate its contents to align with the philosophical and theoretical principles of personhood and person-centred practice as set out in the definition.

By making explicit the philosophical principles of a person-centred curriculum, the programme team is confirming the vision, intentions and priorities of the curriculum. To embed person-centredness in the curriculum, these should be cohesively aligned. The curriculum philosophy frames the intended curriculum as detailed in the programme documentation and benchmarks ways of working so that the vision can be realised in how the curriculum is experienced. As identified earlier in this chapter, Dickson et al. (2020) concluded that a healthcare curriculum is person centred when it is co-constructed, transformative, pragmatic and relational. These principles should be evident in how a person-centred curriculum is designed, delivered and evaluated. Activity 3.3 provides the opportunity to unpack what these four principles mean to you before we go on to consider how we might use them to embed person-centredness in curriculum structures.

A useful approach to determining the extent to which the espoused philosophical or theoretical principles are manifest in a curriculum is using a mapping exercise. Curriculum mapping involves positioning programme structures against philosophical principles to demonstrate whether there is alignment and cohesion (Dyjur et al. 2019). The mapping could take the form of a table, mind map or conceptual map. Mapping curriculum structures to the four philosophical principles underpinning person-centred curricula provides insights into the extent to which person-centredness is embedded in a curriculum. This is exemplified in Activity 3.3.

ACTIVITY 3.3

Mapping the Philosophical Principles with the Curriculum Structures

The purpose of this activity is to provide the opportunity for your programme team to map your curriculum against the philosophical principles that are indicative of person-centredness. You will need a facilitator, sticky tape and A4 copies (one for each small group) of the mapping template shown in Table 3.2.

1. Ask participants to organise themselves into small groups.
2. Within each group, review the mapping template which refers to structural aspects of the curriculum (grey rows) and philosophical principles (blue columns). You may wish to add extra rows to include other aspects specific to the context in which you support learning.
3. In conversation with your small group members, complete the template by recording an X if the philosophical principles are evident in each of the programme structures listed. You may also want to record examples to support your decision.
4. Completed mapping grids should be stuck to the wall to form a gallery.
5. Participants should spend a few minutes reviewing the gallery, observing for where there is consensus or variance.
6. The facilitator should lead a discussion based on the following questions.
   - Where is there agreement that structures are aligned with the philosophical principles?
   - Where is there variation and why?
   - What actions (if any) are needed to further embed person-centredness in curricular structures?

(continued)

(continued)

TABLE 3.2   A Mapping Template.

	Philosophical principles			
Curriculum structures	**Co-constructed**	**Relational**	**Pragmatic**	**Transformative**
Curriculum design				
Approaches to teaching and learning				
Assessment practices				
Approaches to programme evaluation and modification				
(Please insert additional aspects)				

Mapping facilitates the tracking of the person-centred golden thread throughout the curriculum structure. It provides a visual representation highlighting the extent to which the philosophical principles are comprehensively and cohesively embedded through structures. In the next section, we will examine how organisational structures can create the conditions for person-centred ways of working that permeate curricular structures.

Creating Organisational Structures for Collaborative, Inclusive and Participative Ways of Working That Support Collective Leadership

The structure of the curriculum should support the creation of thriving communities with opportunities for all to flourish. This reflects the intention of the World Health Organization's people-centred healthcare policies (WHO 2015) and person-centred practice as advocated by McCance and McCormack (2021). Our view of healthcare practice is therefore a broad concept, encapsulating our values and ways of working with others regardless of context, i.e. as an academic in a university or college, as a facilitator of learning in a healthcare organisation, as a practitioner, as a service provider or as a service user. Structure is therefore not confined to the physical environment of universities or health/care organisations, but rather is an open system that supports learners' experiences of person-centredness.

To create these thriving communities, it is important to think about how structures create connections between a range of stakeholders. This may be achieved in several ways: through networking and collaborations; joint contractual appointments; honorary appointments; and partnership working. Such communities are supported by systems of collective leadership and by organisations that offer educators, policymakers and practitioners opportunities for shared learning. The following vignette outlines a structure of shared governance that supports collective leadership in one university in the UK.

VIGNETTE 3.1

The organisational structure in the Divisions of Nursing, Paramedic Science, Occupational Therapy and Arts Therapies at Queen Margaret University, Edinburgh in Scotland adopts shared governance. This approach is one way in which we put into practice our values and collaborative commitments. Each member of the Division is a member of one of three Shared Governance Groups: Teaching and Learning Delivery and Enhancement Group (TALDEG), Innovations and Partnerships Group (IPG) and Research and Development (R&D). The groups provide a divisional structure for decision making and collaborative working. This approach developed from a desire to move away from a hierarchical management style and towards more collaborative working and shared responsibility or collective leadership. The ways of working have been refined over the past three years and each group has evaluated its progress against strategic objectives and devised new objectives for the next three years. Each Governance Group reports into the Divisional Council that meets five times per academic year and of which all staff in the Division are members. The Governance Groups and Divisional Council have Co-Convenors, a role which is rotated amongst members with each Co-Convenor serving for six months at a time.

A shared governance model of operational management and leadership such as this is an approach that is consistent with person-centred values and principles. It rejects hierarchical models of management and leadership and instead operates a collective model of leadership that sees all team members as leaders and equally accountable for the effectiveness of processes. The approach to working is well established in many healthcare environments internationally but is less well developed in academic settings, where hierarchical approaches continue to dominate.

Central to curriculum structure are of course shared values, explored more fully in Chapter 5. However, espousing what are claimed to be the ideals of person-centredness does not mean that these ideals are lived in everyday activities and actions. Further, others may not experience person-centredness. Engaging in methods of working that are consistent with person-centredness enables all persons to have a 'voice'. Moreover, these ways of working create structures that enable all stakeholders to contribute to shaping the curriculum. They enable a more inclusive, participative and collaborative team, valuing individual strengths and talents within a mutually respectful environment. The following methodologies are implemented to support the collective leadership in the vignette.

- *Habermas' theory of 'communicative action' (Habermas 1981)*: with a focus on interrupting perceived norms through critical, respectful and reflective questioning; working towards intersubjective agreement about ideas and the language used; showing mutual understanding (recognition) of individual perspectives and views; and striving for unforced consensus about what to do in different situations. This is evident in weekly forums and discussion spaces following Divisional Council meetings where colleagues identify a contemporary topic and share understandings and raise critical questions. By identifying critical questions, key actions can be mutually agreed and planned.

■ *Critical creativity (McCormack and Titchen* 2006*)*: blends being critical with being creative to increase potential for our own and others' flourishing that is visible to others (Titchen and McCormack 2010). This is evident in using imagery to create shared ways of working in teams, using collage to evaluate the curriculum and share experiences with others. By engaging in critical creativity and evaluating the process of learning, educators are equipped to use such methods with learners to help them articulate what they know and challenge their assumptions. It is also evident in sharing 'champagne moments' where individuals share their significant achievements, acknowledged in a framed certificate hung on the wall in the Division.

■ *Theory U (Senge et al.* 2005*)*: this theory is underpinned by transformational principles derived from phenomenology. Theory U starts from a basis of 'respect' for all persons and their interpretation of the world. No interpretation is the 'right' one, but individual interpretations of reality influence the nature of one's being and thus how each person behaves in different situations. At the core of Theory U is presencing – sensing and being present. Presencing requires attention to one's being in a situation, sensing feelings in these situations and working to understand. Everybody having responsibility for presencing means they are individually accountable for how they react/respond. It is through critically reflective engagement that individual and collective requirements for change and, ultimately, transformation are identified. In Theory U, change is not a linear process but instead involves five stages that take us through a process of deep reflection, understanding and action – underpinned by the requirement that 'we need to unlearn in order to learn'. Example activities are each member of the department being a member of a triad. In each triad, individuals bring issues and are helped to reflect on the situation and enabled to take action through facilitation. Learning through this process develops facilitation skills. Theory U is also used to evaluate the creation of a healthful culture at different points in time which has raised consciousness about individual contributions and opened discussions around how to strengthen the culture.

These integrated methodologies have been realised through several methods that have been increasingly owned by the whole team, reviewed annually and refined to continue to shape ways of working. All these methods have been underpinned by an operational plan delivered through integrated objectives for which responsibility is held by the different shared governance groups. Progress towards achievement of these objectives is reported to the Divisional Council.

Creating the Conditions for Effective Partnership in Curriculum Review and Design

Working in partnership with a range of stakeholders may feel obvious. Many organisations have stakeholder or advisory groups or councils with the aim of co-design, co-delivery and co-evaluation of curriculum. The intention of such stakeholder groups, according to Virgolesi et al. (2014), is creating collaborative, communicative spaces conducive to authentic co-design, delivery and evaluation.

Simonsen and Robertson (2013) suggest that co-design is a means by which agency of persons in the design of technologies and practices has the intention of transforming workplaces. It features a participatory approach that contributes to workplace democracy. However, consideration of who key stakeholders are, their interest and purpose in the curriculum is important. Stakeholders, including university and practice educators, students, strategy and policy leaders, regulators or commissioners and recipients of healthcare, may all have a contribution to make and in some countries stakeholder engagement is regulated by law. In Norway for example, boards at different levels in universities and university colleges are obligated to have broad representation from various stakeholders. Having this as part of the fabric of organisations gives opportunities to prepare and engage stakeholders to work as equals in these processes. Having structures at all levels can influence the development of modules/units/courses and consider how to achieve the curriculum intentions. Stakeholders may also be involved in how departments are organised in terms of structures to deliver the curriculum, how to include student and stakeholder engagement and processes to meet the intended regulatory requirement and quality standards.

It is important to identify all stakeholders that should be included in the different processes. The identification of which stakeholders to include is dependent on the intended outcome. The outcome may be concerned with the development of modules/units/courses to achieve the curriculum intentions or how to create stakeholder engagement structures to facilitate a person-centred learning environment. Consideration therefore also needs to be given to methods of engagement. For example, you may want to facilitate interactive workshops or discussions or use interactive technologies to encourage learner involvement; use social media to engage learners with current issues or perhaps particular methods of evaluation like Guba and Lincoln's (1994) fourth generation evaluation, which invites participants to engage with claims, concerns and issues about a particular module or other topic for evaluation.

Learners are one type of stakeholder but if they are to contribute meaningfully, they need help in developing their confidence and skills in articulating their views (Dickson et al. 2020). According to O'Donnell et al. (2022), this needs to be facilitated so learners are empowered to participate in the shared governance of educational programmes. Offering support for learner representatives to develop these skills reflects a democratic rather than a bureaucratic approach in the governance of programmes and organisations. If learners are to have a meaningful presence in the governance structure, they need to perceive that their input is not just tokenism but is a meaningful contribution to decision making in partnership with other stakeholders. Dickson et al. (2020) suggest the prerequisites for effective shared governance are that all members role model person-centredness and demonstrate the principles of person-centred practice.

The following vignette outlines structures to involve students at one university in Norway.

VIGNETTE 3.2

At the University of South-Eastern Norway (USN) each class elects two students to be their class representatives to represent them in the Student Council, thus taking part in the Student Democracy which is the student organisation at USN. The class representatives represent the students and work together with lecturers, support staff and other student representatives to improve the experience of current and future students, academically and socially. Class representatives are the link between the students and USN staff, and between the students and the Student Democracy, thus guarding students' interests. Class representatives are responsible for leading class meetings once a month to inform the class about any issues they might have. This enables the class to discuss these. The views of the class are then brought to relevant staff and to the Student Council. The Student Council includes all the class representatives in a faculty and is led by the Student Council President. Class representatives must attend meetings with the Student Council once a month. Furthermore, according to Norwegian jurisdiction, it is required by law that students have a 20% right to representation in all decision-making bodies at Norwegian universities, thus assuring student inclusion at the macro-system level. Additionally, at the national level the Norwegian Agency for Quality Assurance in Education (NOKUT), an independent expert body under the Ministry of Education and Research, annually maps the student experience through a national student survey.

You will notice from the Norwegian example the multiple structures that facilitate student representation so that students have their voices heard and their perspectives and experiences captured across university platforms. The formality of university structures acknowledges the value of the student voice and commitment to using it to drive positive change. This is only one university example. You will be able to think of other examples in other universities and in practice.

The following activity invites you to engage with a webinar before considering how your curriculum is structured to enable students and other learners to contribute to the curriculum.

ACTIVITY 3.4

Mapping Opportunities for Student Representation in the Curriculum

Advance HE in England has a range of resources that promote student voices in the curriculum. Watch the following six-minute Advance HE webinar, 'The Future of the Student Voice. Policy, Principles, Practice' www.youtube.com/watch?v=gVdgaGo61gA.

Now take time to consider the structure within your own context and think about the spaces you create to engage with students.

Map the level of student representation in the different committees within your school/faculty, from course-specific committees to school executive committees.

Remember to consider how the student voice is heard in relation to all aspects of learning, wherever it takes place.

Stakeholders have varying degrees of power and influence over the curriculum. The extent of their vested interest in the curriculum is also variable. Stakeholders may have high power/influence and high interest in the curriculum and therefore would be fully engaged in the process. They may, however, have high power/influence but low interest. Irrespective of their capacity to commit to the process, their level of engagement may increase if an issue of particular interest arises. Some stakeholders may have low power/influence and high interest, such as preceptors and mentors. However, their contribution will also be valuable in supporting students in clinical practice. They may be able to influence more powerful stakeholders, e.g. service users who represent the voices of other service users may influence the involvement of senior managers. It is therefore important to provide all stakeholders with the opportunity to indicate their preferences about the extent and ways in which they wish to be kept fully informed while not feeling overwhelmed by the frequency, volume or relevance of information shared.

When collaborating with stakeholders, a good way of understanding their perspective is to talk with them. Asking them about their views is often the first step in building a successful relationship with them. It is helpful to know what is important to them; what success would look like for them; how they would like to be involved; and how they would like you to communicate with them. To help you consider your stakeholders, you may wish to engage in the following activity.

ACTIVITY 3.5

1. This is a group activity. The purpose is to identify key stakeholders who will work together to achieve a specific curriculum outcome.
   - Consider the people who will be affected by what you are doing/trying to achieve.
   - To begin, identify each stakeholder on a post-it note.
   - Discuss the needs of each stakeholder and their interest in the curriculum.
   - Consider their level of influence and their vested interest and identify this on the power/interest grid below.
   - Place the post-it note for each stakeholder on the relevant part of the grid.

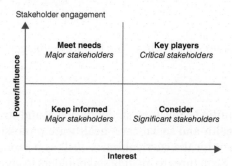

2. Ascertain how engaged are they with the current programme. There are five levels of engagement.

(continued)

(continued)

- Unaware – unaware of the current programme.
- Reluctant – stakeholders are aware of current programme but reluctant to change.
- Neutral – stakeholders are ambivalent and are neither resistant or supportive of the programme.
- Supportive – stakeholders are supportive of the programme.
- Leading – stakeholders are aware of the programme and are currently engaged in promoting the success of the programme.

	Unaware	Reluctant	Neutral	Supportive	Leading
Stakeholder 1					
Stakeholder 2					
Stakeholder 3					
Stakeholder 4					
Stakeholder 5					

3. Identify their current level of engagement and their desired level of engagement with the programme.

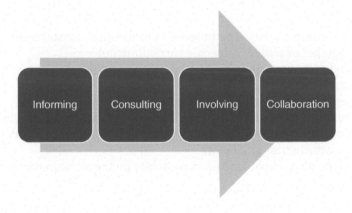

For each stakeholder, identify how you facilitate engagement in the organisation of the programme.

You may have identified educators, students, policy and strategy leaders, recipients of and providers of health and social care, healthcare professionals and leaders from clinical practice relevant for the curriculum, as well as persons from public or private interest organisations. Structures to include stakeholders in co-design could be through participation in stakeholder or practice advisory boards and include workshops or other activities with the intention of creating collaborative communicative spaces conducive to the design of relevant modules/units and courses in the curriculum.

VIGNETTE 3.3

At the University of South-Eastern Norway, representatives from municipal health and care services were invited to explore and discuss competence needs in service provision when developing a new Master's programme in community nursing. This ensured that the programme was relevant for clinical practice and that stakeholders developed ownership of the programme. This was particularly successful for elective courses in the Master's programme, for example the Advanced Nurse General Practitioner programme. Other ways in which stakeholders were included in implementing and evaluating a curriculum included having healthcare workers from clinical practice continually contribute as supervisors in formative and summative assessment development, other assessment methods such as simulation, written assignments and creating other assessments and exams during modules/units/courses as well as discussion and other types of feedback. Another example of a formal collaborative arrangement between practice and educational institutions is where staff hold joint appointments in both places, being 50% at the hospital and 50% at the college/university. This ensures collaboration between the institutions and reciprocal stakeholder engagement. In doctoral education, other stakeholders might include relevant experts in research from other universities or representatives from statutory organisations who may be responsible for allocating funding and/or ensuring quality standards.

The next activity encourages you to think about how you will include stakeholders in meaningful ways. It encourages you to think about the spaces you might construct to ensure appropriate engagement. This will, however, be addressed more fully in the next chapter on systems (Chapter 4).

ACTIVITY 3.6

How to Include Stakeholders in Meaningful Ways

Map out how you currently communicate/engage with all your stakeholders. For each stakeholder, identify how you communicate with them. Is it by newsletter, annual report, email or in various committees? For example, the regulatory Nursing and Midwifery Board of Ireland requires each educational institute to submit an annual report for each programme.

	Annual report	Interactive workshop	Newsletter	Committees	Email	Social media
Stakeholder 1						
Stakeholder 2						
Stakeholder 3						

(continued)

(continued)

- In your curriculum group, reflect on how you can make your communication/engagement strategies with your stakeholders more meaningful and interactive.
- How adequate are these structures in engaging stakeholders you have identified using the grid?
- What other structures will you need to create to engage with all stakeholders?
- Within these structures, how will you meaningfully involve all key stakeholders?
- How might you gain the interest of people who are not immediately supportive or manage their opposition?
- What are the consequences of stakeholder involvement/non-involvement?

Creating Spaces to Promote Learner Autonomy So Learners can Participate Fully in Person-centred Curricula

As the intention of person-centred curricula is transformative, traditional teacher-directed learning methodologies will not create the conditions that make this possible. Such approaches do not privilege relationships or encourage active participation in co-construction. An inclusive curriculum that promotes student autonomy aims to avoid excluding some learners, thus promoting a person-centred curriculum. Stentiford and Koutsouris (2022) describe an inclusive curriculum as one that recognises all learners and makes learning accessible to all learners. The framework of the Universal Design for Learning (UDL), originally developed by CAST (www.cast.org/impact/universal-design-for-learning-udl), supports the development of an inclusive curriculum as it facilitates diversity of content, assessment and teaching strategies. The three core principles of the UDL are multiple approaches to engagement; many forms of representation; and multiple actions and expressions. The curriculum structure is key to enabling learner-centred approaches. This can often be viewed as a challenge because of the learning contexts such as the classroom and other learning spaces, limitations of timetabling and the increasing reliance on the use of virtual learning environments. These constraints also offer opportunities for innovation.

Recognising learners as autonomous and respecting that their previous life experience and culture influence how they see the world are hallmarks of person-centred curricula. Creating spaces to encourage learners to learn from each other and to value the experiences of their fellow students and help learners to understand their own learning needs meets the prerequisites of the curriculum. Offering choice in learning can be framed by helping learners set their own learning objectives but the learning culture needs to foster participation, inclusivity, mutual respect and collaboration between learners (Dickson et al. 2020).

There is mounting pressure on educational institutions to increase the number of undergraduate healthcare professional students. Educational institutions are required to identify the maximum number of students they can facilitate in providing safe learning spaces and high-quality programmes. Learning environments may be constrained by organisational factors, privileging pragmatic solutions. The lack of physical space may mean online teaching is the only choice for educators. Due to a shortage of placements, the UK Nursing and Midwifery Council (NMC) allows students to have up to a maximum of 600 hours simulated learning, which may seem at odds with person-centred learning that occurs in real-life situations where students learn from their interactions with healthcare professionals and their clients. In person-centred curricula, autonomy is valued and therefore finding innovative ways of engaging with students can be achieved.

The next activity encourages you to identify spaces that can support person-centred TLA.

ACTIVITY 3.7

Identifying Spaces for Learning

Consider the availability of spaces to support person-centred learning activities.

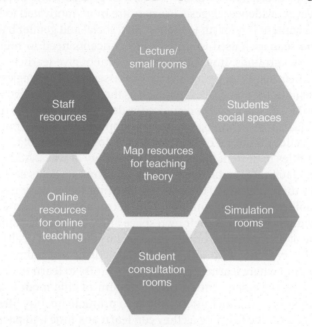

GROUP WORK OR SMALL GROUP TEACHING

- Identify the resources you need to support person-centred learning activities.
- Identify the supports required to support person-centred online education.
- Identify the supports required to facilitate simulation.

SIMULATED LEARNING

- Brainstorm on how to develop person-centred scenarios for simulation.
- Identify the prerequisites to support person-centred learning in a simulation environment.

LEARNING IN CLINICAL PRACTICE

- What supports are required to support clinical accessors (preceptors or mentors)?
- What is the maximum number of students that can be facilitated on each placement at a particular time?

Being innovative requires recognition that learners have preferences in the way they wish to learn and curricula providing flexible options to engage with learners can be responsive and flexible to individual need. Structures that support recognition of prior learning can provide flexible options for entry to programmes. Promoting choice is one way of promoting student engagement. This choice may be in the form of optional modules, optional clinical placements or opportunities to do some modules or placements abroad, for example Erasmus programmes. While on their programmes, learners have different preferences for their optimal method for presentation of information. Some learners may prefer visual or auditory forms of information rather than printed text. There are specific guidelines for the presentation of written information to facilitate accessibility by all. Learners may prefer to learn in groups while others may prefer to learn solo. However, evidence suggests learners are more motivated to learn if they can identify how the content is relevant to their ethnic, social and gender background. Thus, reading lists and scenarios used to explain key concepts need to reflect the diversity of the learners' backgrounds. Innovations in assessment give learners different options to demonstrate their learning. Using a variety of assessment strategies, such as essays, MCQs and presentations, practical exams such as the OSCE (Objective Structured Clinical Examination) foster creativity and choice for demonstrating skills or knowledge.

Interactive learning technologies are also opportunities for innovative teaching and learning practices. The use of learning technology such as Blackboard or Canvas creates opportunities to present information in a variety of ways. Additionally, learning technologies can facilitate interactive learning and thus students can receive immediate feedback on their progress. However, all learning technology needs to adhere to relevant accessibility guidelines. Online modules can also offer learners flexibility and facilitates individuals to learn at their own space and at a time that suits them.

An example of an innovative online module, targeted for all healthcare professionals, is 'Making Every Contact Count'. This module consists of online content followed by a skills workshop where learners have an opportunity to learn their new skills using role play. This fosters person-centred care. The aim of this module is to educate all healthcare professionals on brief interventions to promote healthy lifestyles.

Learners value online learning as they can learn at a time and pace that suit themselves. The next activity invites you to consider online learning options and whether they best represent a person-centred curriculum.

ACTIVITY 3.8

Online Learning

Identify the different types of online learning that are available to your students. How many of the activities are student centred?

1. List the programmes which include an online component, followed by a workshop. One example would be the Crisis Prevention Intervention programme. This aims to educate healthcare professionals to respond to crisis situations with a focus on prevention, using verbal de-escalation skills and strategies where restraint is inappropriate.

2. List the online programmes which are mandatory for students and registered staff. Examples include an infection control programme available in HSeL, an an online platform for healthcare professionals in Ireland (www.hseland.ie), and the NHS elearning hub (www.e-lfh.org.uk).

3. Some students may like to learn from service users. The following are two Massive Open Online Courses (MOOCs), co-developed with service users and are freely available.
   - Improving Health Assessments for People with an Intellectual Disability (www.futurelearn.com/courses/health-assessment).
   - Women's Health After Motherhood (www.futurelearn.com/courses/womens-health-after-motherhood).

Curriculum structure helps to keep learners engaged with the programme. Having clear information about submission dates and timelines for progression on programmes provides structure for progression. However, person-centred curricula offer flexibility to support learners who require extensions on submission dates or need to defer placements. Flexibility in structure can allow learners to rejoin at a later date. Learners who require extra support, such as those with learning or physical disabilities, can receive this to facilitate them completing the programme. Learners who have specific needs, such as learning disability or physical illness, may require extra support while on placements. The following vignette gives an example of how learners with disabilities are supported in one university.

VIGNETTE 3.4

All students in TCD (Trinity College Dublin) are advised to register their disability, be it physical or learning or other disability, when they commence their studies. The disability officer will assess the individual needs of each student and agree reasonable accommodations in partnership with clinical assessors. Reasonable accommodation is any action that helps to alleviate a substantial disadvantage due to a disability and/or significant ongoing illness. All undergraduate students are also allocated a tutor, an academic who provides support and advocacy to their allocated students. Tutors work in partnership with the disability officer to advocate for reasonable accommodation for their students.

Examples of reasonable accommodation include the following.

- Additional time for assessments or to learn specific skills.
- Assistive technology.
- Human/personal supports (such as note-takers, readers, Irish Sign Language interpreters, etc.). For health professions, personal assistance is considered appropriate provided that the individual's knowledge and skill are assessed, rather than those of the assistant.
- Information in alternative formats.
- Physical access to required areas and/or timetabling of course elements into accessible locations.
- Alternative forms of assessment.
- Alternative or specifically selected practice education experiences that enable the student to demonstrate core competences in an environment with fewer barriers.

ACTIVITY 3.9

Please review the resources on UDL.

- https://udlguidelines.cast.org/?_gl=1*1qzsmoq*_ga*OTA5OTA4ODgxLjE2OT I1NDEzMjM.*_ga_C7LXP5M74W*MTY5MjYwNjQwMC4zLjEuMTY5MjYwNj Q0NS4wLjAuMA.

Take the quiz to ascertain if your current teaching practice adheres to the principles of UDL.

- https://ahead.ie/Dara/udlscore/story_html5.html

ACTIVITY 3.10

- Reflect on how you can incorporate the framework for UDL in your curriculum.

Giving learners optimal flexibility in terms of what, when and how learning is organised promotes their autonomy and self-determination and ultimately person-centredness (O'Donnell 2021; Cook et al. 2022). This flexibility needs to be cognisant of the learning organisation requirements and registration bodies accrediting programmes. The following activity encourages you to consider the flexibility/rigidity of your programme.

ACTIVITY 3.11

1. Where in your programmes are there opportunities to foster flexibility for learners?
2. Do your programmes allow students to plan parts of their own learning, for example design what units of study they might pursue?
3. Where can learners access exchanges in learning environments?
4. Can learners choose where to do their practice learning (within the accreditation requirements)?
5. Is flexibility promoted for entry into the programme?
6. Is learner choice promoted in the assessment strategy?
7. Is the programme flexible to meet the additional needs of learners (deferral of practice learning opportunities or assessments, helping learners to take time out of the programme, etc.).

SUMMARY

- Structure refers to spaces at multiple levels across the curricular system and also in programme design, by laying out a pathway for how programmes are organised to facilitate and assess learning in sequential ways.
- A focus on structure seeks to introduce and consolidate learning while embedding humanistic values to inform ways of being and doing. The person-centred practitioners we seek to develop will be heard in practice, but they need space to voice their thoughts, feelings, ideas and learnings and model their behaviours and associated actions in a supportive curriculum.
- Curriculum structure is therefore fundamental to creating cultures of transformation. A structure that is embedded in person-centred principles and values creates the conditions for collective leadership and shared responsibility of the curriculum and offers opportunities to embed the four philosophical principles of the Person-centred Curriculum Framework.
- Creating spaces for stakeholder involvement and ongoing evaluation promotes curricula that are flexible and responsive.

REFERENCES

Brand, G., Sheers, C., Wise, S. et al. (2021). A research approach for co-designing education with healthcare consumers. *Medical Education* 55 (5): 574–581.

Cook, N., Brown, D., O'Donnell, D. et al. (2022). The Person-centred Curriculum Framework: a universal curriculum framework for person-centred healthcare practitioner education. *International Practice Development Journal* 12 (Suppl): 1–11.

Dickson, C., van Lieshout, F., Kmetec, S. et al. (2020). Developing philosophical and pedagogical principles for a pan-European person-centred curriculum framework. *International Practice Development Journal* 10 (Suppl. 2): 1–20.

Dyjur, P., Grant, K., and Kalu, F. (2019). *Curriculum Review: Curriculum Mapping*. Taylor Institute for Teaching and Learning. Calgary: University of Calgary.

Guba, E.G. and Lincoln, Y.S. (1994). Competing paradigms in qualitative research. *Handbook of Qualitative Research* 2 (163–194): 105.

Habermas, J. (1981). *The Theory of Communicative Action* (trans. T. A. McCarthy). Boston, MA: Beacon Press.

McCance, T. and McCormack, B. (2021). The person-centred practice framework. In: *Fundamentals of Person-centred Healthcare Practice* (ed. B. McCormack, T. McCance, C. Bulley, et al.), 23–40. Chichester: Wiley Blackwell.

McCormack, B. and Titchen, A. (2006). Critical creativity: melding, exploding, blending. *Educational Action Research* 14 (2): 239–266.

O'Donnell, D., McCormack, B., McCance, T. and McIlfatrick, S. (2020). A meta-synthesis of person-centredness in nursing curricula. *International Practice Development Journal*, 10, Special Issue on Person-centred Curricula, Article 2.

O'Donnell, D., Dickson, C., Phelan, A. et al. (2022). A mixed methods approach to the development of a person-centred curriculum framework: surfacing person-centred principles and practices. *International Practice Development Journal* 12 (Suppl): 1–14.

Senge, P., Sharmer, C.O., Jaworski, J., and Flowers, B.S. (2005). *Presence: An exploration of profound change in people, organizations, and society.* New York: Random House.

Simonsen, J. and Robertson, T. (ed.) (2013). *Routledge International Handbook of Participatory Design.* London: Routledge.

Stentiford, L. and Koutsouris, G. (2022). Critically considering the 'inclusive curriculum' in higher education. *British Journal of Sociology of Education* 43 (8): 1250–1272.

Titchen, A. and McCormack, B. (2010). Dancing with stones: critical creativity as methodology for human flourishing. *Educational Action Research* 18 (4): 531–554.

Virgolesi, M., Marchetti, A., Piredda, M. et al. (2014). Stakeholders in nursing education: their role and involvement. *Annali Di Igiene (Annals Of Hygiene)* 26 (6): 559–569.

Willis Commission (2012). Quality with Compassion: The Future of Nursing Education. Report of the Willis Commission on Nursing Education. williscommission.org.uk.

World Health Organization (2015). Global Strategy on People-centred and Integrated Health Services. Interim Report. Geneva: WHO.

CHAPTER 4

Systems

> This chapter begins by exploring the 'systems' component of the Person-Centred Curriculum Framework. Systems within the teaching, learning and assessment (TLA) methods are used to achieve curriculum outcomes. The chapter aims to align connections from strategy, structure and systems to help learners focus on the desired assessment outcomes. To do this, we invite you to draw explicitly on educational/pedagogical theories related to adult (professional) learning, considering how to include this in the education of healthcare professionals. We dare you to challenge traditional systems to 'let go' of old ways of doing and being. Finally, we provide a variety of activities to help you think critically about the systems component of the Person-Centred Curriculum Framework in your organisations and how it can foster the flourishing of person-centredness in healthcare professionals.

INTRODUCTION

This chapter focuses on the systems component of the Person-Centred Curriculum Framework. The Person-Centred Curriculum Framework promotes a system focused on approaches to TLA that explicitly articulate the philosophical principles of personhood and enable flexibility in programme delivery. Key to person-centred TLA methods are educators and leaders who are committed to embodying the values of person-centredness and adopting an overarching facilitative approach to their practice. A Person-Centred Curriculum Framework involves integrated systems that (i) promote focused approaches to TLA that explicitly articulate the philosophical principles of personhood; (ii) facilitate flexibility in programme delivery; (iii) develop educators and leaders who are committed to embodying the values of person-centredness; (iv) support

Developing Person-Centred Cultures in Healthcare Education and Practice: An Essential Guide, First Edition. Edited by Brendan McCormack.
© 2024 John Wiley & Sons Ltd. Published 2024 by John Wiley & Sons Ltd.

educators and leaders to adopt an overarching facilitative approach to their practice; and (v) utilise facilitated learning and assessment strategies as core to TLA.

Philosophical Principles Underpinning the Systems Component of the Person-centred Curriculum Framework

Within the framework of our person-centred curriculum, systems are described as 'learning and assessment methods used to achieve the stated curriculum outcomes'.

This chapter explains how the philosophical principles of the Person-centred Practice Framework of McCormack et al. (2021) were applied in developing the systems component of the Person-Centred Curriculum Framework. The Person-centred Practice Framework has significantly impacted the field of person-centeedness worldwide and helps to develop a person-centred culture that benefits healthcare professionals and patients (see Chapter 2 for a detailed overview of the framework). The framework also helps to recognise the complexity within healthcare systems and expresses the dynamic character of person-centredness. It provides a framework for learning, leadership, clinical practice and research by providing a common language and shared understanding and a system of person-centred practice.

The Person-Centred Practice Framework comprises five domains.

- Macro-context (which focuses on the strategic and political factors that influence the growth of person-centred culture).
- Prerequisites (which focuses on staff characteristics).
- Practice environment (which focuses on the environment in which healthcare is provided).
- Person-centred processes (which focuses on ways of engaging that are required to establish connections between people).
- Outcome (which focuses on the outcomes of effective person-centred practice) (McCance and McCormack 2021).

This chapter will focus on the first and third domains, Macro-context and Practice environment (meso-context), in the context of the Person-Centred Curriculum Framework.

The macro-context reflects the strategic and political factors that influence the development of person-centred cultures. It operates at both the individual and collective levels; thus, individual educators must constantly be reflective and conscious of their teaching approaches and how they can be influenced by the socio-political context in which they work (Baldie et al. 2021; McCormack et al. 2021). The development of person-centred health systems and the Person-Centred Curriculum Framework is influenced by the macro-context in which healthcare or education is provided. Socio-political dynamics are present throughout healthcare systems, at all organisational levels, among healthcare professionals and between healthcare professionals, patients and their families (Baldie et al. 2021).

In the Person-centred Practice Framework, four key socio-political influencing factors sit within the macro-context: (i) health and social care/policy frameworks, (ii) strategic frameworks, (iii) workforce developments and (iv) strategic leadership. These attributes operate regionally (within the country), nationally, internationally and globally (Baldie et al. 2021; McCormack et al. 2021).

1. *Health and social care/policy frameworks*: guidelines for the creation and assessment of person-centred cultures at the international, national and local levels, along with their vision, mission and time frames.
2. *Strategic frameworks*: a visionary plan that illustrates how the organisation's strategic goals relate to developing person-centred cultures and are supported by its many activity programmes.
3. *Workforce developments*: it takes a lot of work and many different strategies, policies and programmes to train and maintain a healthy healthcare work environment that can meet the present and future needs of person-centred cultures.
4. *Strategic leadership*: a practice where executive leaders create a vision and utilise various management, leadership and influence techniques to assist organisations and teams in adapting to prosper in the face of rapid technological and economic change.

The practice environment reflects the complexity of the context in which healthcare is experienced. The position taken in the Person-centred Practice Framework is that context is synonymous with the practice environment, and contained within it are multifaceted characteristics and qualities of the environment (people, processes and structures) that impact the effectiveness of person-centred practice. Attributes of the practice environment include (i) appropriate skill mix; (ii) shared decision-making systems; (iii) effective staff relationships; (iv) power sharing; (v) physical environment; (vi) supportive organisational systems; and (vii) potential for innovation and risk taking (McCormack et al. 2021).

1. *Appropriate skill mix*: staffing levels and diversity regarding knowledge and skills necessary to deliver high-quality, context-specific services.
2. *Shared decision-making systems*: organisational dedication to teamwork that emphasises open communication and mutual respect.
3. *Effective staff relationships*: to provide comprehensive, person-centred cultures, effective interpersonal relationships are essential.
4. *Power sharing*: pursuing the best possible outcomes for both parties by committing to shared values, aims, aspirations and desires rather than exploiting others.
5. *Physical environment*: healthcare facilities strike a good aesthetic-to-practical balance by prioritising design, privacy, sanctuary, choice/control, safety and universal access to serve patients, their families and healthcare professionals.
6. *Supportive organisational systems*: organisational systems that encourage initiative, creativity, independence and personal safety, supported by a governance framework that emphasises culture, relationships, values, communication, professional autonomy and accountability.

7. *Potential for innovation and risk taking*: practising professional accountability in decision making that balances the best available facts, professional judgement and local information.

The systems component of the Person-Centred Curriculum Framework supports environmental/organisational structures, processes and administration, creating a systems world that supports the lifeworld in realising purpose. The philosophical dimension used in the systems component is pragmatic, and methodological principles are built on a philosophy of pragmatism. TLA strategies are pivotal in establishing an educational system that integrates theory and practice seamlessly. They provide a platform for constructive debate, allowing learners to analyse idealism versus realism critically. Enquiry-based learning enables learners to navigate complex, multi-layered contexts effectively. Learning experiences are situated within the dynamic interplay of local, national and global perspectives. Encouraging the generation and sharing of diverse evidence sources supports the development of competence (knowledge, skills and attitudes).

Furthermore, TLA strategies empower learners to perceive themselves as catalysts for social change. They promote an ethos of comfort with complexity, fostering resilience in the face of intricate challenges. TLA strategies also promote continuous evaluation of the learning process in terms of the learning environment and pedagogical methods. They create communicative spaces that facilitate social learning and the construction of meaning, enabling safe spaces to evolve into environments conducive to courageous discourse. Ultimately, these strategies enable learners to grasp the relevance of person-centred practice through contextualised, real-life learning experiences.

These TLA strategies offer a multifaceted approach to enhancing the educational system, emphasising the integration of theory and practice, critical discourse and development of socially conscious, competent learners.

There needs to be a whole-system understanding of person-centred healthcare with the following factors.

- Whole-system thinking.
- Creation of communicative/learning spaces.
- Provision of transparent (resource and material) frameworks.
- Set person-centred healthcare in alignment with other/similar perspectives.
- Boundaries removed.
- Frontline staff and learners' experiences used as major evaluation criteria of whole-system quality.
- Managing resources (practice environment).
- Understanding the challenges in practice (practice environment).
- Staff knowledge and skills, including academic and clinical (prerequisites)

This comprehensive approach ensures a well-rounded exploration of person-centred healthcare within the broader healthcare system.

ACTIVITY 4.1

OBJECTIVE

To facilitate an activity that helps participants develop a comprehensive understanding of person-centred healthcare within a whole-system context, focusing on key elements such as whole-system thinking, communicative spaces and transparent frameworks.

MATERIALS NEEDED

Whiteboard or flipchart and markers, printed copies of the provided suggestions and examples, and small group discussion materials (optional).

INSTRUCTIONS

1. Introduction (15 minutes)
   Welcome participants and introduce the activity's objective: to explore and understand person-centred healthcare within a whole-system context. Explain the importance of a holistic approach to person-centred care.
2. Whole-system thinking (20 minutes)
   Discuss the concept of whole-system thinking and its significance in person-centred healthcare. Use the whiteboard or flipchart to illustrate key points and engage participants in a brief discussion.
3. Group activity – creating communicative spaces (30 minutes)
   Divide participants into small groups (if the group is large) and provide each group with a printed copy of the suggestions and examples for creating communicative/learning spaces. Instruct each group to brainstorm and outline a plan for creating communicative spaces within their healthcare settings. Encourage creativity and innovation.
4. Group sharing – communicative spaces (15 minutes)
   Reconvene as a large group and invite each small group to share their ideas and plans for creating communicative spaces. Facilitate a brief discussion around each shared idea, allowing participants to ask questions or provide insights.
5. Transparent frameworks (20 minutes)
   Discuss the importance of providing transparent frameworks in person-centred healthcare. Highlight how clear resource and material frameworks can enhance the delivery of care. Engage participants in a discussion about the challenges and benefits of transparent frameworks.
6. Boundary removal and alignment (20 minutes)
   Explain the concept of removing boundaries and aligning person-centred healthcare with other similar perspectives or approaches. Use examples to illustrate how alignment can improve overall healthcare quality.

(continued)

(continued)

7. Evaluation and reflection (20 minutes)
   Discuss the role of frontline staff and learners' experiences as major evaluation criteria for whole-system quality. Encourage participants to reflect on their experiences and how they contribute to evaluation in their healthcare settings.
8. Conclusion (10 minutes)
   Summarise the key takeaways from the activity, emphasising the importance of whole-system understanding in person-centred healthcare.

This activity will give participants a deeper understanding of person-centred healthcare within a whole-system context. By exploring concepts such as whole-system thinking, communicative spaces, transparent frameworks and alignment with other perspectives, participants will be better equipped to contribute to and enhance person-centred care in their professional roles.

A supportive meso-/macro-context is essential for advancing person-centred healthcare. This context should encompass elements such as incorporating service design thinking, well-defined guidelines for implementing person-centred care, a culture of openness to feedback, organisational alignment with person-centred values, and effective recruitment and retention strategies.

ACTIVITY 4.2

OBJECTIVE

To engage participants in a creative and interactive challenge to build a supportive meso-/macro-context for person-centred healthcare, emphasising innovation, teamwork and out-of-the-box thinking.

MATERIALS NEEDED

Whiteboard or flipchart and markers, printed copies of the provided suggestions and examples, and art supplies (markers, sticky notes, poster boards).

INSTRUCTIONS

1. Introduction (15 minutes)
   Welcome participants and introduce the activity's objective: to explore and develop a supportive organisational culture for person-centred healthcare. Explain the significance of a supportive meso-/macro-context in promoting person-centred care.

2. Service design thinking brainstorm (20 minutes)
   Start with a session where participants brainstorm how service design thinking can enhance person-centred care. Encourage them to use markers and sticky notes to jot down their ideas on a designated 'innovation wall' or whiteboard.
3. Guideline development challenge (30 minutes)
   Form teams of participants and challenge each team to develop a set of guidelines or criteria for implementing person-centred healthcare within their organisation. Provide art supplies and poster boards for teams to represent their guidelines visually. Set a timer to add an element of urgency.
4. Guideline gallery walk (15 minutes)
   Allow each team to present their visual guidelines to the group in a 'gallery walk' style. Encourage teams to explain their creative choices and concepts.
5. Open communication artefacts (20 minutes)
   Instruct participants to create visual artefacts (e.g. posters, infographics or illustrations) that symbolise open communication and organisational values supporting person-centred care. These artefacts should be imaginative and expressive.
6. Recruitment and retention innovation (30 minutes)
   Challenge participants to brainstorm and design innovative recruitment and retention strategies using art supplies. Teams should create visually appealing representations of their strategies.
7. Solution showcase (15 minutes)
   Have each team present their recruitment and retention innovations, highlighting their creative approaches. Encourage teams to inspire each other with their out-of-the-box ideas.
8. Conclusion (10 minutes)
   Conclude the challenge by summarising the key takeaways and emphasising the creative solutions generated.

   This creative challenge transforms the discussion of person-centred healthcare into an interactive and engaging experience. By incorporating art and teamwork, participants are encouraged to think creatively and collaboratively, leading to fresh ideas and solutions for building a supportive meso-/macro-context in their healthcare organisations.

Thematic Actions

The thematic actions identified from the systems component of the Person-Centred Curriculum Framework offer ideas for teams to consider within their organisation. Below are shown thematic actions highlighting some key indicators of the systems component of the Person-Centred Curriculum Framework. Perhaps there are even more ways in which the systems component is congruent with person-centred approaches and philosophy in the educational environment (Table 4.1).

TABLE 4.1   Thematic actions of the systems component of the Person-centred Curriculum Framework.

- Support educators in becoming person-centred facilitators of the workplace and work-based learning and assessment.
- Draw explicitly on educational/pedagogical theories related to adult (professional) learners' learning with consideration given to how to include this in the education of professionals.
- Offer multiple/alternative assessment methods per programme to offer choice while still achieving learning outcomes.
- Ensure connections from strategy, structure and systems to assessment are aligned to help learners focus on the outcomes.
- Create safe reflective spaces throughout programmes to enable learners to explore their personhood.
- Develop opportunities for learners to be immersed in realistic practice environments (such as simulation, living labs, etc.) to enable authentic learning.
- Co-design (university/practice) assignments foster shared values, understanding and commitment.
- Develop a system supporting learners' ownership of their own learning.
- Monitor learning and progress with developmental tools such as learning analytics and individualised and consistent mentorship.
- Emphasise the effectiveness of arts-based and creative methods to connect people with their personhood.
- Dare to challenge traditional systems to 'let go' of old ways of doing and being.

FREQUENTLY ASKED QUESTIONS ABOUT THE SYSTEMS COMPONENT OF THE PERSON-CENTRED CURRICULUM FRAMEWORK

What is the System?

Systems that support the development and delivery of a Person-Centred Curriculum Framework should align the TLA methods with the curriculum outcomes, explicitly articulating the philosophical principles of personhood (McCormack and McCance 2017). A person-centred approach reflects the principle of co-construction and requires flexibility, offering choices for learners and supporting them in understanding their own learning needs concerning person-centred practices (Cook et al. 2022; Gaebel et al. 2018; Dickson et al. 2020). Educators and leaders committed to embodying person-centredness through facilitated learning and assessment strategies are key to the person-centred TLA method. They encourage multi-stakeholder assessments and portfolios where learners can use creativity to demonstrate their learning. The systems supporting ownership of learning include developmental tools such as learning analytics to monitor learning and progress (Cook et al. 2022).

Learners should also have individualised and consistent coaching and mentorship. Creating safe, reflective spaces throughout programmes enables learners to explore their personhood (Cook et al. 2022). This is fundamental to cultural humility, whereby learners critically reflect on their values, beliefs and assumptions in shaping their worldview and interacting with others (Cook et al. 2022; Sanchez et al. 2019). Creating spaces for reflection and critical dialogue is core to person-centredness and requires experienced facilitators of learning to help learners make sense of their experiences.

ACTIVITY 4.3

OBJECTIVE

Embark on an exciting journey to uncover the intricate web of systems that support person-centred education and learning. This immersive and interactive expedition will allow participants to understand and experience the dynamic interplay of these systems.

MATERIALS NEEDED

Large open space or room with movable furniture, coloured yarn or string, art supplies (markers, coloured paper, stickers, sticky notes), printed copies of the provided suggestions and examples, and small group discussion materials (optional).

INSTRUCTIONS

1. Introduction (15 minutes)
   Welcome participants to the 'Person-Centred Learning Ecosystem Expedition' and explain the objective: to explore and experience the complex systems supporting person-centred education. Set the adventurous tone by sharing a brief story or metaphor about embarking on a journey of discovery.
2. Creating the ecosystem (30 minutes)
   In the centre of the room, place a large poster or board labelled 'Person-Centred Learning Ecosystem'. Provide participants with coloured yarn or string and instruct them to choose a specific aspect or system from the suggestions and examples. Encourage participants to attach one end of their yarn to the central ecosystem poster and move to different parts of the room to represent different systems. As participants connect their yarn to various systems, they are visually creating a dynamic ecosystem.
3. Group exploration (40 minutes)
   Divide participants into small groups (if the group is large) and assign each group a different aspect of the person-centred learning ecosystem. Instruct each group to visually represent their assigned system on a large piece of coloured paper.
4. Ecosystem showcase (20 minutes)
   Invite each group to showcase their visual representation of a specific system to the entire group. As each group presents, ask them to explain how their system contributes to person-centred education and its interconnectedness with other systems.
5. Experiential exploration (30 minutes)
   Transitioning to experiential stations around the room represents a different aspect of the person-centred learning ecosystem. Participants can engage in activities or discussions at each station to gain firsthand experience and insights into these systems. For example, one station might involve role-playing

(continued)

(continued)

as educators embodying person-centredness, while another could explore assessment methods that support individualised learning.

6. Reflective dialogue (20 minutes)

Gather participants for a reflective dialogue in a circle. Facilitate a discussion on the following topics.

- What did you discover during this ecosystem expedition?
- How did embodying person-centredness play a role in your journey?
- What connections did you observe between different systems within the ecosystem?
- What creative insights can be applied to enhance person-centred education in your context?

7. Interactive mind map (15 minutes)

Use sticky notes and markers to create an interactive mind map on a whiteboard or poster. Participants can contribute their key takeaways and ideas by placing sticky notes on the mind map.

8. Conclusion (10 minutes)

Conclude the expedition by summarising the key discoveries and insights made during the journey.

This immersive expedition allows participants to delve into the intricate web of systems that support person-centred education while engaging their creativity and experiential learning. It transforms learning into an exciting adventure, leaving participants with a profound understanding of the interconnectedness of these systems.

Why is the System Important in the Curriculum, and How is it Implemented?

The systems component of the Person-Centred Curriculum Framework is important because it helps create a person-centred environment and culture that supports educators in becoming person-centred facilitators of the workplace and work-based learning. To make educators autonomous, decisions on how to carry out their subject and move away from traditional lectures need to be made (Cook et al. 2022). Educators are prepared through appropriate programmes and work alongside experienced facilitators, enabling them to find their style of facilitating learning (Gaebel et al. 2018). They use various methods, including flipped classrooms, hybrid classrooms and simulated and social learning opportunities. This allows the educators to be immersed in realistic practice environments alongside learners (such as simulation, living labs, etc.), enabling authentic learning. The curriculum offers multiple/alternative assessment methods that offer choice while still achieving learning outcomes. Learners should co-design assessments, thereby fostering shared values, understanding and commitment. The systems component creates safe reflective spaces throughout programmes, enabling learners to explore their personhood.

ACTIVITY 4.4

In this interactive activity, participants will delve into the significance of the systems component of the Person-Centred Curriculum Framework and explore practical strategies for its implementation. Through group discussions, brainstorming and hands-on activities, participants will better understand how this component can foster a person-centred educational environment.

MATERIALS NEEDED

Whiteboard or flipchart, markers, sticky notes and printed curriculum framework excerpts.

INSTRUCTIONS

1. Introduction (15 minutes)
   Begin the activity by providing an overview of the importance of the systems component in the Person-Centred Curriculum Framework. Emphasise its role in creating a person-centred culture in education.
2. Group discussions (20 minutes)
   Divide participants into small groups and assign each group one aspect of the systems component, such as educator autonomy, diverse teaching methods, authentic learning environments, alternative assessments and safe reflective spaces.
3. Exploration and brainstorming (30 minutes)
   In their small groups, participants should explore their assigned aspect in more detail. Use printed excerpts from the curriculum framework to provide context. Encourage each group to brainstorm practical strategies and ideas for implementing their assigned aspect effectively.
4. Group presentations (30 minutes)
   Each group presents their findings and implementation ideas to the entire activity. Encourage creativity and use of visuals to make the presentations engaging.

EXAMPLE PRESENTATION

Aspect: Diverse teaching methods
Presentation format: Role-play and interactive discussion
Content:

- Role-play scenario: participants demonstrate a traditional lecture-style teaching approach.
- Interactive activity: participants then engage in a flipped classroom exercise, demonstrating how this method immerses learners in realistic practice environments.

(continued)

(continued)

  ▪ Discussion: discuss the benefits of diverse teaching methods, highlighting how the flipped classroom approach aligns with person-centred principles.
5. Collaborative brainstorming (15 minutes)
   After all presentations, reconvene as a whole group. Engage in a collaborative brainstorming session to identify common themes and overarching strategies for implementing the systems component.
6. Action planning (20 minutes)
   Based on the identified strategies, encourage participants to develop action plans to incorporate the systems component into their educational practices. Each participant should outline specific steps, timelines and resources needed.
7. Conclusion (10 minutes)
   Conclude the activity by facilitating a reflective discussion. Ask participants to share their insights and commit to implementing at least one strategy discussed during the activity. Provide ongoing support and follow-up to help participants implement the strategies and monitor their progress.

This activity offers a dynamic and collaborative way for participants to explore the importance of the systems component and develop practical strategies for its implementation. It engages educators, administrators and curriculum developers in a collective effort to create a person-centred educational environment.

How Would We Know If Our System Was Successful?

The system's success may also be measured by how well it facilitates the collaborative curriculum design that fully and coherently incorporates person-centred principles and ideas into the theoretical and practical frameworks during the planning and development stages. The main success metric is how well the curriculum aligns with the organisational system to help educators deliver the curriculum as intended. This requires a system that encourages active participation and teamwork among stakeholders aware of and committed to their roles and responsibilities in promoting person-centred education and practice.

ACTIVITY 4.5

In this creative and interactive activity, participants will embark on a quest to measure the success of the person-centred curriculum system in a fun and engaging way. This quest will involve collaborative problem-solving, role-playing and creative challenges to assess how well the system aligns with person-centred principles and encourages stakeholder teamwork.

MATERIALS NEEDED

Envelopes with quest challenges (prepared in advance), whiteboard or flipchart, markers and sticky notes.

INSTRUCTIONS

1. Introduction (10 minutes)
   Set the scene by explaining that participants are embarking on a quest to evaluate the success of the person-centred curriculum system. Emphasise that they will encounter challenges related to person-centred principles and collaboration.
2. Form questing teams (5 minutes)
   Divide participants into teams, ensuring a mix of roles and responsibilities (educators, curriculum designers, administrators, learners) in each team.
3. Quest challenges (40 minutes)
   Provide each team with a series of sealed envelopes containing quest challenges. Each challenge should be related to assessing different aspects of the curriculum system's success. Challenges can include riddles, scenarios or creative tasks.
   Example quest challenges:
   - 'The Alignment Enigma': solve a riddle to find evidence of alignment with person-centred principles in the curriculum documentation.
   - 'Collaboration Conundrum': role-play a scenario where stakeholders must collaborate to design a person-centred course.
   - 'Learner's Labyrinth': create a visual representation of the learner's journey through the curriculum, highlighting person-centred elements.
4. Quest completion (30 minutes)
   Teams open their envelopes, one at a time, and work together to complete the challenges. They should discuss, brainstorm and be creative in their responses. Use a whiteboard or flipchart to display the progress of each team as they complete challenges.
5. Group discussion (15 minutes)
   Gather all participants for a group discussion. Each team presents their findings and solutions for the quest challenges. Encourage teams to explain how their responses reflect the success or areas of improvement in the person-centred curriculum system.
6. Conclusion (10 minutes)
   Lead a reflective discussion on the insights gained during the quest. Ask participants to reflect on the importance of person-centred education and teamwork in curriculum design. Invite participants to commit to taking specific actions or initiatives based on the quest's outcomes. Conclude the activity by celebrating

(continued)

(continued)

the successful completion of the quest. Encourage participants to carry forward the lessons learned during the quest into their real-world efforts to enhance the success of the person-centred curriculum system.

This interactive quest activity makes the evaluation process engaging and enjoyable and fosters a deeper understanding of the importance of person-centred principles and collaboration in curriculum design. It encourages participants to actively explore and reflect on the curriculum system's success playfully and creatively.

Unpacking System Themes

The thematic actions serve as a framework for examining the systems component, the nexus connecting TLA methods to achieve predefined curriculum objectives. This framework also advocates for focused pedagogical approaches that explicitly articulate the philosophical principles underpinning the concept of personhood. The system should facilitate adaptability in programme delivery, enabling educators and leaders to embody the core values of person-centredness. These thematic elements provide educators and leaders with a comprehensive facilitative approach to their professional practice (Table 4.2).

SUMMARY

- Promote focused approaches to TLA that explicitly articulate the philosophical principles of personhood.
- Person-centred staff support system (for educators and leaders) in various forms (ALS, buddies, etc.), facilitated by person-centred ambassadors.

TABLE 4.2   Activities to illustrate the practical implementation of these thematic actions within the systems component.

- Creating safe spaces for working with creativity.
- Applied drama work, sympathetic presence.
- Portfolio assessment that includes summative and formative assessment.
- Critical creativity work.
- Facilitation and behaviours (Michelle Hardiman facilitation).
- Della fish.
- Peer learning: learners design their own assessment strategies (describe the method, steps and stages).
- Fishbowl as a mechanism.
- Flipped classroom.
- Technology, including simulation (high and low fidelity).

- A larger mix of teaching and learning methods: flip the classroom, online learning management systems (e.g. Canvas), software to foster groups, online engagement for social learning, hybrid classrooms, e-modules, blended learning, simulated learning and assessment within practice contexts/skills labs.
- Unambiguous frameworks and student coaching allow learners to balance a desire for predictability/certainty while navigating a flexible and uncertain programme/ curriculum and meeting assessment criteria.
- Flexibility and adaptability to enable change with change/need in society.
- Support session, in practice, using reflection, directly related to person-centred practice and what is required to provide person-centred education and develop person-centred practitioners.
- Foster a person-centred physical learning environment.

REFERENCES

Baldie, D., McCance, T., and McCormack, B. (2021). Sociopolitical context in person-centred practice. In: *Fundamentals of Person-centred Healthcare Practice* (ed. B. McCormack, T. McCance, C. Bulley, et al.), 159–168. Oxford: Wiley.

Cook, N., Brown, D., O'Donnell, D. et al. (2022). The person-centred curriculum framework: a universal curriculum framework for person-centred healthcare practitioner education. *International Practice Development Journal* 10 (Suppl 4): 1–20.

Dickson, C., van Lieshout, F., Kmetec, S. et al. (2020). Developing philosophical and pedagogical principles for a pan-European person-centred curriculum framework. *International Practice Development Journal* 10 (Suppl 4): 1–20.

Gaebel, M., Zhang, T., Bunescu, L., and Stoeber, H. (2018). *Learning and Teaching in the European Higher Education Area*. Brussels: European University Association.

McCance, T. and McCormack, B. (2021). The person-centred practice framework. In: *Fundamentals of Person-centred Healthcare Practice* (ed. B. McCormack, T. McCance, C. Bulley, et al.), 23–32. Oxford: Wiley.

McCormack, B. and McCance, T. (ed.) (2017). *Person-centred Practice in Nursing and Health Care: Theory and Practice*, 2e. Chichester: Wiley Blackwell.

McCormack, B., McCance, T., and Martin, S. (2021). What is person-centredness? In: *Fundamentals of Person-centred Healthcare Practice* (ed. B. McCormack, T. McCance, C. Bulley, et al.), 13–22. Oxford: Wiley.

Sanchez, N., Norka, A., Corbin, M., and Peters, C. (2019). Use of experiential learning, reflective writing, and metacognition to develop cultural humility among undergraduate students. *Journal of Social Work Education* 55 (1): 75–88.

CHAPTER 5

Shared Values

In this chapter, we begin by considering what is meant by shared values in the context of a person-centred curriculum. We will explore how agreeing and making shared values explicit is core to benchmarking ways of being among all those who influence or experience person-centred healthcare education. As in other chapters, we invite you to engage in a series of activities designed to clarify individually held values and values that are shared by others in your team and learning organisation. We will consider how shared values influence what we and who we prioritise, how we interact with others and how we support learning. Together, we will explore how shared values are exemplified and nurtured through inclusive and collaborative learning cultures where person-centredness and human flourishing are experienced.

INTRODUCTION

This chapter focuses on the shared values component of the Person-centred Curriculum Framework. Shared values are fundamental to the effective operation of a complex system (Waterman et al. 1980), including healthcare education (McCormack et al. 2022). For this reason, in an illustration of the seven elements of a healthcare education system, McCormack et al. (2022) situated shared values as central to the operation of the complex system (Figure 5.1).

Shared values should be mutually agreed by members of a team or department and validated as the basis for ways of being and working. Changes in shared values are likely to have major implications for the dynamics and effectiveness of the overall complex system. In considering person-centredness in healthcare curricula, co-creating shared values forms the basis for open and transparent processes of engagement. Having shared values creates a frame of reference in relation to expectations, approaches and standards of behaviours (Manley et al. 2014). The team's shared values should be

Developing Person-Centred Cultures in Healthcare Education and Practice: An Essential Guide, First Edition.
Edited by Brendan McCormack.

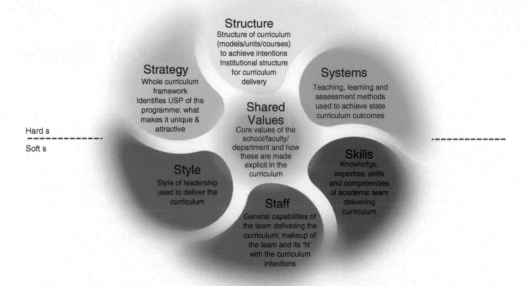

FIGURE 5.1   Visual representation of the seven elements of a healthcare education context.
Source: McCormack et al. (2022, p. 6)/with permission of Sage Publications Inc.

aligned with the professional framework and regulatory Code of Conduct specific to the respective disciplines represented in the team.

In developing the Person-centred Curriculum Framework, a set of five thematic actions was identified to shape how shared values influence the effective functioning of a team and contribute to the development of a healthful learning culture (O'Donnell et al. 2022). The thematic actions are shown in Table 5.1. These five actions highlight fundamental considerations in agreeing and embedding shared values in a

TABLE 5.1   Thematic Actions (Shared Values).

1. Identify specific ways of being person centred in approaches and attitudes to students and colleagues (fostering healthful cultures); role modelling reciprocal respect and understanding during working and learning relationships.
2. Promote reciprocal and authentic interest in the lifeworld of other persons, see them as 'owners' of their own lifeworld, and then co-create from the shared/blended lifeworlds.
3. Make values explicit. Encourage conversations about the importance of values and creating healthful cultures.
4. Provide opportunities for shared decision making and active participation using consensus and/or spaces to create shared purposes and interpretations of a person-centred curriculum.
5. (Co-)translate discussions to ensure the language of the curriculum framework is meaningful, recognisable and understandable to the various users (academic, clinical, stakeholder and learner perspectives), and explicitly linked through local policies, documents and concepts.

Source: Adapted from O'Donnell et al. (2022, p. 9).

person-centred curriculum that is delivered across a range of academic and clinical learning environments. This chapter will explore how the thematic actions can be implemented to agree and embed shared values across the whole team that is engaged in supporting learning so that person-centredness is consistently prioritised and role-modelled irrespective of where learning occurs.

FREQUENTLY ASKED QUESTIONS ABOUT SHARED VALUES

What are Shared Values?

In the context of the Person-centred Curriculum Framework, shared values are defined as:

> The core values of the school/faculty/department and how these are made explicit in the curriculum.
>
> *(McCormack et al. 2022, p. 6)*

The definition establishes a connection between people's shared professional values and how these are demonstrated through the curriculum. Where a curriculum is authentically person centred, the value of personhood should be evident in the strategies, structures, systems, staff, skills and leadership styles of those who influence and experience the curriculum. In this context, shared values should not be assumed or imposed but rather should be negotiated in collaboration with all those who have a vested interest in or affiliation with a specific learning programme (curriculum). Values in a person-centred curriculum focus on building and sustaining relationships with others while appreciating their uniqueness and potential as persons. The core values of person-centred practice such as mutual respect, self-determination and negotiated autonomy (McCormack et al. 2021) may be considered when the team is formulating its shared values. However, the shared values should be unique to the team and negotiated until consensus is reached so that the values are meaningful and relevant to the persons involved in a particular learning context.

In a person-centred curriculum, the shared values should be expressed in a way that reflects an intentional focus on working together with, rather than on, persons. The team should agree specific ways of being person centred in their approaches and attitudes to others, including learners and colleagues who support academic and practice learning. All persons involved in the curriculum should have their voices heard. In turn, they should role model reciprocal respect and understanding in their working and learning relationships so that experiences are quality assured as person centred and healthful. The shared values should enable the identification of agreed expectations and outcomes for everyone so that priorities and acceptable ways of working are explicit, understood and owned by all.

Why are Shared Values Important in Curricula?

The critical reason why shared values are important is because they create the learning culture in which a curriculum operates. When values are shared among members of a programme team and are visible and experienced by others engaged in the curriculum, then person-centredness becomes the ethos of the programme (O'Donnell 2021). Shared values privilege experiences and outcomes that the people engaged in the curriculum have identified as important to them. In this way, shared values create the conditions for transformation by empowering others and enabling flourishing and well-being. By agreeing shared values among those who influence or engage in a person-centred curriculum, there is a commitment to honouring and upholding personhood as the threshold concept underpinning ways of being, acting and becoming.

By implication, pedagogical approaches should also be aligned with the team's shared values. For example, person-centredness may be achieved by using socially just, inclusive and flexible pedagogies that embrace diversity and well-being, creating a healthful learning culture (O'Donnell 2021). Where person-centredness is reflected in a team's shared values, relationships become grounded in an appreciation of personhood and the uniqueness, contributions and potential of all persons. Having shared values creates the foundations for cohesive teamwork, collective endeavour, a strengths-based approach and the conditions for ethical and innovative practice.

How Would We Know If Values are Shared Among the Learning Support Team?

When shared values are embodied in the practice of individual team members, there will be congruence between what is espoused (what the team agreed their shared values to be) and behaviours lived out in practice (where actions are aligned with and exemplify the shared values). However, shared values can also be evidenced when team members hold themselves accountable by challenging each other when their practice is inconsistent with the agreed values. Approaches to doing this, by having a courageous conversation, are explored later in this chapter.

There are many other ways in which shared values can be evidenced in a curriculum and in approaches to learning, for example through the curriculum philosophy; when there is a focus on personhood; when facilitation and active learning approaches are used to optimise dialogue and engagement; and through inclusive, participative approaches. Where decision making is shared, relationships are collaborative, leadership is transformational and innovative practices are supported, then person-centredness is in operation (McCormack and McCance 2017).

UNPACKING KEY THEMES (THEMATIC ACTIONS)

A primary consideration in promoting person-centredness is recognising the necessity of creating learning cultures where person-centredness is experienced. McCormack (2022) highlights that to achieve person-centredness, culture must be developed and sustained by people who espouse the principles and values of person-centredness that are also manifest in organisational values and systems. Without experiencing and working in person-centred ways, person-centredness becomes conceptual and intangible to learners, educators, practitioners and those in our care. In acknowledging the necessity of a healthful culture for person-centred learning, we recognise that an important initial consideration involves clarifying our values and agreeing an explicit shared purpose to develop the culture. Mutuality, or a shared purpose, exists when those in the organisation or team align their values with their vision. This is the foundation of successful change as it creates meaning and incentive to strive for something that transcends each team member but can be achieved together.

Activity 5.1 is a reflective exercise that provides the opportunity to reflect on your values and how these are manifest in your approaches to supporting learning.

ACTIVITY 5.1

In this activity you are encouraged to complete the worksheet below by reflecting on your values and how they influence your teaching and learning practices. You should complete questions 1–5 of the worksheet by yourself and then meet to discuss it with a colleague or supervisor to agree actions to align values with approaches to supporting learning.

WORKSHEET

The purpose of this worksheet is to help you to reflect on your own professional values to better understand how they are evident in your educational practice and interactions with others at work. This exercise may also make you more aware of situations when you believe you are not living up to your values, why that may happen and what you could do differently in future. Please work your way through the worksheet by answering each question in the space provided.

Date of individual reflection (Questions 1–5 completed): _____

1. The three most important professional values I have are:
   _____
   _____
   _____

2. My values are aligned with person-centredness because: _____
   _____

3. In relation to living up to my values in how I support learning, what I have learned is:
   _____

4. The thing that stands out for me about others' professional values is:
   _____

5. The most important thing I have learned about supporting learning in a person-centred healthcare curriculum is:
   _____

   Date of meeting with colleague: _____
   Colleague/supervisor's name: _____

   (continued)

(continued)

ACTIONS AGREED AT MEETING WITH COLLEAGUE

My actions (prior to my next meeting with my colleague/supervisor) to align my values and practice with person-centred ways of being are to:

_____

_____

_____

_____

SUMMARY

The summary can be added to over time as you continue to reflect on your values and the ways in which these are demonstrated in how you support learning.

My values	How I demonstrate my values in supporting learning as part of a person-centred curriculum
_____	_____
_____	_____
_____	_____

Source: Adapted from Dewing et al. (2014, p. 27).

SHARED LANGUAGE

As introduced in Chapter 2 (Strategy), central to the development of shared values is the ability to communicate effectively using language that successfully conveys an intended message. For this to occur, language needs to be unambiguous and culturally sensitive. Additionally, where person-centred approaches to education, learning and practice are espoused, language should also be indicative of the core values of personhood which demonstrate mutual respect, authenticity, autonomy and self-determination (McCormack et al. 2021). Activity 5.2 builds on the exercises from Chapter 2 and further highlights some language considerations, this time in relation to supporting learning. Let us think about the language we use in our learning organisation and consider how it aligns (or not) with person-centred values.

ACTIVITY 5.2

We invite you to complete the template below by identifying types of language that you feel should be avoided in professional healthcare education. For each example, please record your rationale for avoiding this wording and offer a person-centred

Language to avoid	Rationale for avoiding	Person-centred alternative wording
The student		
Non-achiever		
Cohort effect		
Early leaver		

alternative. Some examples are provided but you can include further examples of your own by adding additional rows.

The purpose of this activity is to reflect on the language that we use and how the choice of words may or may not be aligned with person-centred values. Language, whether written or spoken, is a powerful instrument in conveying messages regarding what is or is not valued. Vygotsky (1986) contended that concepts become meaningful in the way that they are verbally communicated and that having a shared appreciation of language serves as a tool to express understanding. Language may explicitly or implicitly reveal attitudes that are communicated to others in healthcare practice (Goddu et al. 2018). Similar findings have been confirmed in educational contexts. O'Donnell (2021) found that students who had experience of a person-centred curriculum were sensitised to the use of language. They reported that the use of terms which reflected the value of personhood created an affiliation with clinical staff who learners perceived as having similar values. Language may therefore be interpreted as an expression of a person's values. Manley et al. (2014) identified that shared values form a mutual frame of reference that helps create the parameters for establishing belonging, support and self-direction. These concepts are critical to effectively supporting learning.

In relation to person-centredness in healthcare education and practice, an issue that is commonly reported is the interchangeable use of terminology (Leplege et al. 2007; Miles and Asbridge 2014; Harding et al. 2015). There is ongoing debate about how concepts such as person centred, patient centred, client centred, family centred, student centred and learner centred are defined and the extent to which they are similar or can be differentiated. Klancnik Gruden et al. (2021) acknowledged the potential for conceptual overlap and concluded that literature relating to a range of concepts may be of relevance to discussions about person-centredness. McCormack et al. (2021) definitively clarified that the key conceptual distinction between terms is that person-centred practice applies equally to all persons and embraces all the core values of person-centredness (McCormack et al. 2021). It is argued that by focusing on a specific role or person, some persons are being privileged over others which is contentious in upholding the equity and autonomy of all persons. Using the term 'person centred' overcomes this challenge.

What Language Do You Use in Your Curriculum?

Language challenges may be particularly evident when the learning context involves an international audience and persons who use different primary languages. One example is the use of the word 'flourishing' which, while common parlance in English, can create tensions for educators in other countries who may be challenged to find a directly comparable term. An awareness of the use and meaning of language is relevant to all learning settings where barriers may be created by using a range of other factors such as clinical terminology or generalisations that may be demeaning or exclusive. This highlights the importance of never assuming that meaning is understood as language is open to translation and interpretation not only across disciplines, cultures and countries but depending on each person's knowledge, experience and capacity to assimilate that which is communicated. It is also possible that even where language is understood in words, meaning may be obscured due to differences in its interpretation.

CREATING PERSON-CENTRED LEARNING CULTURES

The extent to which there is congruence between espoused shared values and behaviours observed in practice is a key indicator of workplace culture. At its simplest level, culture is commonly understood as 'how things are done around here' (Drennan 1992, p. 9) and reflects the social context that influences the way people behave (Sanders et al. 2021). A concept analysis undertaken by Manley et al. (2011) identified the essential attributes to describe an effective workplace culture, which are presented in Table 5.2.

TABLE 5.2 Essential Attributes of an Effective Workplace Culture.

1. Specific values promoted in the workplace, namely:
   - person-centredness
   - lifelong learning
   - high support and high challenge
   - leadership development
   - involvement, collaboration and participation by stakeholders
   - evidence use and development
   - positive attitude to change
   - open communication
   - teamwork
   - safety (holistic).
2. All the above values are realised in practice, there is a shared vision and mission and individual and collective responsibility.
3. Adaptability, innovation and creativity maintain workplace effectiveness.
4. Appropriate change is driven by the needs of patients/users/communities.
5. Formal systems (structures and processes) to continuously enable and evaluate learning, evaluation of performance and shared governance.

Source: Manley et al. (2011, p. 9).

Building on this work, Sanders et al. (2021) identified a framework of four 'guiding lights' focusing on how to recognise and develop effective workplace cultures that are also good places to work.

- Collective leadership.
- Living shared values.
- Safe, critical, creative learning environments.
- Change for good that makes a difference.

In this framework, each guiding light is clearly described and aligned to intermediate and ultimate outcomes which are reflective of healthful workplace cultures.

Exploration of culture in the context of agreeing shared values is central to the development of healthful workplace cultures. There is a range of tools that can be used to examine workplace culture, such as the Workplace Critical Culture Analysis Tool (WCCAT) (Wilson et al. 2020), which is an observational tool aligned directly to core concepts within the Person-centred Practice Framework (McCormack and McCance 2017). When focusing on a systems-level approach to person-centredness in healthcare curricula, as is the case when using the Person-centred Curriculum Framework, it is important to identify who will take forward any culture change work, their ability to influence at different levels and their transformational leadership qualities, including expert facilitation skills. Exploring culture and context is addressed in greater detail in Chapter 7. However, as a starting point, Activity 5.3 provides an opportunity to reflect on the connection between shared values and their impact on your workplace culture.

ACTIVITY 5.3

We invite you to consider the essential attributes of an effective workplace culture presented in Table 5.2. Can you identify evidence of how each element is, or is not, present in your current workplace? What does this tell you about the shared values that are prioritised within the team in which you support learning?

Creating a No Blame Culture

No blame climates are central to living out person-centred values in learning situations. Such a climate is fundamental to how we work together to remain solution focused and person centred. Being solution focused is when we cognitively engage in positive principles and practices to construct solutions to a challenge/problem, rather than focusing on the problem. In doing so, we acknowledge the challenge but put our energy into the solution rather than remaining stagnant by focusing negatively on the challenge. In this way, we create momentum to move forward. Furthermore, when we begin to explore our learning culture and the values that underpin it, we are often faced with an awareness of values that are not ideal and do not live up to person-centred ways of being and working. This is part of being human. We may not always reach our aspirations and goals and we may perceive that we have failed. However, by adopting a growth mind-set, we can learn from such experiences and strive to move forward. In our journeying, our goal is to narrow the gap between the ideal values and actual values. This requires us to be open to giving and receiving feedback, being solution focused and constructive. Our emotional intelligence and maturity will be key factors here and this requires a climate of valuing each other, acceptance and high support alongside high challenge. Blame cultures do not facilitate this.

A prerequisite to providing a person-centred curriculum is a facilitative culture. This requires us to explore our culture to understand it and establish mutuality to develop it further. Understanding and developing culture is a key skillset for leaders and facilitators of change as it is about the social contexts that influence how people think and behave and therefore the socially expected and accepted norms (Manley et al. 2011). If we are seeking to bring about change, an inevitable part of working and growing in any organisation or team, we need to be able to comprehend why people think, feel and behave the way they do in relation to learning and development. Developing learning cultures therefore starts with values clarification, a shared mission statement and philosophically aligned leadership approach. Agreeing these foundational principles influences the culture that is created and embodied. It is also essential to acknowledge that more than one culture may operate within an organisation where micro-teams exist. Cultures may vary according to the context, commitment and engagement within and between these groups. In such situations, culture change can be particularly challenging, as experiences of culture are likely to be nuanced. However, it also means that culture change can happen at local team levels, giving rise to opportunities to create positive change that radiate outwards.

In education and healthcare organisations where learning happens, we need to consider the learning culture, that is the culture experienced by learners but also by those who facilitate, support and shape their learning. In healthcare education, we also need to consider all the areas within which students learn. In this regard, it is not just the culture of the education institution but also the culture in healthcare settings where students learn in practice, alongside the culture of those organisations that influence both practice and education (e.g. policy makers, professional regulators). We therefore are often working within and across a macro-level system of subcultures and units of organisation. This requires us to bring people together in different forums to create a shared vision for learning that will facilitate person-centredness to be lived out authentically through mutuality irrespective of where learning occurs.

AGREEING PRINCIPLES OF ENGAGEMENT

An example of how to take forward your values is to co-create an agreed set of principles for the team to work with. At the School of Nursing and Paramedic Science at Ulster University, work was undertaken to achieve this. A safe space was created for team members to consider to what extent we were living out our shared values. We identified principles of engagement to frame our ways of being. The principles are used to supportively challenge ourselves and each other at moments when our behaviours appear not to be aligned with our shared values. The steps taken to agree the principles of engagement are as follows.

1. We used an online tool (Padlet™) to facilitate staff to anonymously make preliminary entries about principles of engagement. This approach fostered a psychologically safe space for staff to articulate their views about the principles based on both the good practice and challenges they had experienced. In tandem, the same process was undertaken with learners. Class representatives facilitated engagement with 1400 undergraduate students to capture their views.
2. The principles were then reviewed collectively and integrated into a set of draft principles of engagement. The draft was shared with the academic, technical and business support staff, and the student population, for consideration and revision.
3. At a school retreat, the draft principles and feedback were shared. Team members were asked to individually review and suggest amendments to the draft. The same process was completed with learners through a Student Voice event. Feedback was collated.

Figure 5.2 presents the endorsed principles of engagement which are centrally displayed in the department and shared with all new staff and students.

VALUES CLARIFICATION

The purpose of the next exercise (Activity 5.4) is to provide some ideas about how to raise the profile of values and beliefs in your team/organisation and create the opportunity for dialogue. This is an important step in preparing to develop a mission statement and shared vision. It is through the application of the values and mission statement that we can begin to bring about a culture change. However, to move beyond rhetoric, in addition to having shared values and a mission statement, culture change will only happen where there is also effective leadership and collective action.

Undertaking Activity 5.4 will help your team/organisation to focus on working towards a person-centred learning culture by illustrating how core values and beliefs affect how we work together (including with students) and adopting a no-blame climate. This exercise will assist the team in undertaking an evaluation that explores ideal values (those people say they have) and those that are lived out in the practice of supporting learning. It also facilitates us in recognising where the ideal and actual values are in harmony, while also highlighting those that do not align in order that they can be worked upon.

Engaging in a Values Clarification Exercise

This first step begins by clarifying beliefs and values, being respectful of what emerges through this process. There are various activities that can support us to become aware of and distil our values. An easy initial activity is to ask your team to start recognising

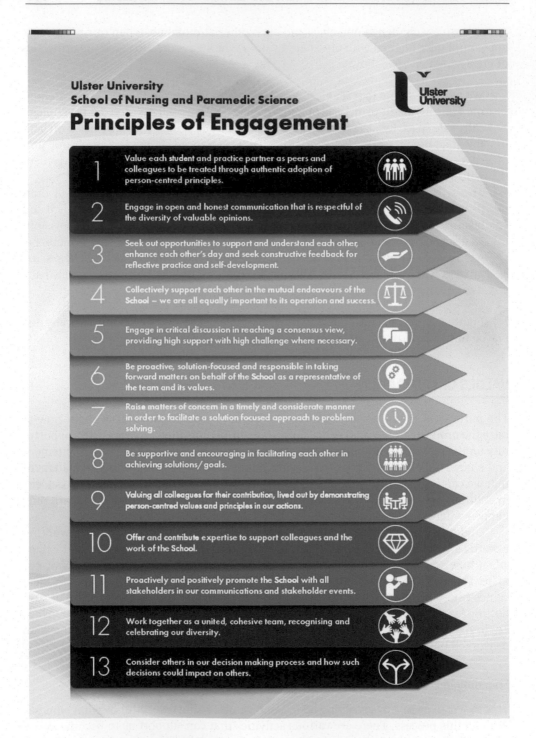

FIGURE 5.2   Principles of engagement.

when values and beliefs are being lived out and openly express this at different moments through your working relationships, including when you are working with different stakeholders. This can bring to life values and beliefs, rather than them being concepts on a poster or set out in a charter. Point out kindly when you see certain values in an interaction or intervention, in what someone says or does not say. Constantly remind yourself and others that when we expose our values to each other like this, we are going to honour and respect each other. While we do this, we should avoid being judgemental but remain reflective and considerate. It is not about taking someone down or selectively building someone up, but about elevating the way we work with each other that is consistently respectful, supportive and empowering.

ACTIVITY 5.4

A Team's Values Clarification Exercise

This is a formal activity, starting off with individual work (preparation), followed by group work. Proficient facilitation skills are necessary to carry out this activity. The five questions to be answered by this exercise are:

- What is the purpose of person-centredness in healthcare curricula?
- How can this purpose be achieved?
- What are the factors that help us achieve this purpose?
- What are the factors that hinder us in achieving this purpose?
- What other values and beliefs do we hold that are important to us?

 STEP 1: GETTING READY

You will need to bring people together to undertake this activity, so plan a date, time and venue that will maximise attendance. Being as inclusive as possible will produce a more meaningful output. Make sure that people know the purpose of the activity before they come, its importance and what it relates to. For example, you could state in the invite:

> This activity is to explore our values and beliefs about person-centred healthcare curricula to start developing shared values and beliefs about person-centred education. If we can develop and agree to a set of shared values and beliefs, we can become clearer about what we do and what we might want to do about delivering the curriculum together. You are asked to contribute as much as you want and to do this as honestly as you can.

(continued)

(continued)

You will need a space where you can put up flipcharts for an extended period (e.g. three weeks) and a flipchart sheet for each of the questions (5) and some sticky notes in five different colours. Each of the flipchart sheets will be hung on the wall or a flipchart stand. Then do the following.

- On the first sheet, create a statement from the first question: for example, I believe the purpose of person-centred healthcare curricula is ...
- On the second sheet, put: I believe this purpose can be achieved by ... and so on.

You may need more than one set of five sheets depending on the number of people you have. Choose five coloured sticky notes. Put a different colour sticky note securely on each flipchart sheet, beside the heading, so you have only one coloured sticky note per question.

STEP 2: RUNNING THE ACTIVITY

Ask each person in attendance to complete the statement (on each flipchart) using a sticky note for each answer they would like to provide. They should not share their responses with others but work autonomously in the first instance. They need to know which colour sticky notes are used on which flipchart sheet. They can provide more than one answer, as long as they are on a separate sheet. You can also do this with technology (such as Mentimeter™ or Padlet), the benefit being that answers go onto each sheet anonymously. Give people time and space to complete each of the five sheets, one by one.

STEP 3: THEMING THE STATEMENTS

Once everyone has completed the activity, it is time to pull these together in themes. This is done as a group exercise and is as inclusive of all the people present as possible. This can be a creative, learning exercise as well as part of work. The most straightforward way to do this is to organise an inclusive group for each of the questions, i.e. five different groups that will theme one question each. The process is then to:

- ask the group to read through the sticky notes and check out the meaning of the statements with each other
- theme the notes on their flipchart sheets and give each theme a short name that accurately represents the content of that theme
- choose short phrases that describe that theme (called attributes or characteristics). They should look for patterns; for instance, they may see that some of the themes seem to link with each other
- advise the group that themes, characteristics and patterns must be supported by what is written on the sticky notes; that is, no new ideas are brought in. They are representing all of the views, not generating new views.

Please note that the group which is dealing with 'Other values and beliefs I con-sider important in relation to' need to review the notes and see which of the other groups the notes can be given to. As the facilitator has oversight, they should support this group. Alternatively, the facilitator(s) can do this theming quickly and suggest which other flipcharts these other values and beliefs sticky notes could be added to.

STEP 4: SHARING THE THEMES AND DRAFTING SUMMARY STATEMENTS

Once this theming has been completed, each group should share their themes with all the participants present. The facilitator again invites any focused comments on what the themes mean, as opposed to an open discussion about themes or whether they are 'correct'. The themes need to remain authentic to the contents of the sticky notes. This can take about 30 minutes, depending on the number of participants and questions being addressed. Remember, there may be some uncomfortable truths emerging and consideration needs to be given to the sensitivity this may bring with it.

As the comments are aired, the facilitator invites comments from the partici-pants on their experience of this activity and highlights any emergent learning points. The themes are refined amongst the discussion and transcribed onto a flip-chart sheet. In doing so, they are written as 'we believe' themes as we have moved from the individual to the collective view.

The aim is to ask each group to write up a draft summary statement that cap-tures concisely their theme and its attributes. This should not be done until the group have clarified what each concept and attribute mean to them, especially if it is a piece of jargon or a buzz term. For example, you could ask: 'What do we mean by high standards?', 'What is effective feedback?' or 'Whose voice?'. Stress again that participants must only work with what they have and any connecting words that are needed, such as 'the', 'and', 'if', 'with', etc.

STEP 5: PUTTING VALUES AND BELIEFS INTO PRACTICE

Once you have the four summary statements (remember the fifth question is merged amongst the others), you will need to help the group decide if others in the team not present need an opportunity to consider the draft values and beliefs and how this will happen. If a consultation is carried out, then you will have a set of shared values and beliefs that people say they have – but this is only the beginning. You now need to consider how to put these values and beliefs into practice. Two questions you can use to facilitate a discussion about this process are:

- How do you expect to see these shared values and beliefs lived out in delivering the curriculum?
- How do you expect gaps between these values and beliefs and our provision to be responded to?

(continued)

(continued)

This is about negotiating with stakeholders how the shared values and beliefs need to be a dynamic presence in how we deliver the curriculum, and what they can expect to happen if they are not used to shape our delivery. Remember, different stakeholders may come with different views on all these elements and so there needs to be authentic collaboration and inclusivity across all these activities.

Once the values and beliefs are established, and an action plan to address any potential gap, you are ready to work on a mission statement.

COURAGEOUS CONVERSATIONS

In living out our values, and in the pursuit of establishing and maintaining shared values, we are sometimes challenged by what we see, hear or experience. These situations are challenging as they often do not resonate with our shared values and to be authentic in our relationships with others, and to ensure we retain or achieve the culture set by these shared values, we need to have courageous conversations. Sometimes it will feel easy to raise the matter, other times it will feel overwhelming. You might feel you are at the bottom of a hierarchy, like you might not be supported by others, or that you might offend or upset the other person, despite your intention to work within agreed values and frameworks. In these situations, we need to draw on our inner strength to take considered action. Koenig (2013) advises that we start with being clear about what we are afraid of saying; often what we are afraid of saying are words we have never spoken before, or at least out loud.

ACTIVITY 5.5

1. Think about a situation you were in when you felt you could not speak up but being true to your values required you to.
2. What was it that you were afraid of saying?
3. Try to write those words down and say them aloud – did this make it feel easier?

Intentions

Often, we avoid courageous conversations because we are afraid matters will become confrontational. Courageous conversations are often about meaningful dialogue, they are not about you being right and someone else being wrong. Once the other person feels they are being pitched as being wrong, they will become defensive and the battle starts. Staying true to the shared values and being explicit that your intentions are honourable and solution focused will encourage the other person to do so too.

ACTIVITY 5.6

1. Thinking about the same situation, when you wrote down what you wanted to say, what was your intention?
2. If your intention was about who is right or wrong, would what you wanted to say have led to meaningful dialogue?
3. Reflecting on this, what could you have said that could have led to meaningful dialogue?

Demonstrating Integrity

In having a courageous conversation, we need to put who we are being to the forefront. Often, the words we say come across differently based on the qualities and values we exhibit when we say them. We need to be prepared to be respectful regardless of how the other person responds and we need to follow through, despite our own anxiety about raising the matter.

ACTIVITY 5.7

1. What are the values you would have most liked the other person to recognise in the situation you reflected on?
2. Thinking of the matter you wanted to raise, how could you exhibit those values?

Having the Conversation

Having thought through your approach and knowing the qualities you want to exhibit, the next step is to bring about the right conditions for the conversation. Koenig (2013) advocates that we use partnering language, whereby the other person is not put on the defensive but is invited to engage in the conversation that will be about you listening as well as getting across your intention. This will need you to consider a suitable time and place to have the conversation and to have a form of words to set the tone and introduce the context of the conversation. An example is: Would you have time for us to explore how we could revisit aspects of this together?

ACTIVITY 5.8

1. Thinking about the same situation, what opening statement/question could you have used to demonstrate partnering language?

Being Attentive

When you have the conversation, remember not to rush. Ensure you have allowed adequate time to think things through beforehand and adequate time to have the conversation; this often takes longer than you might imagine. Take time to pause and consider responses; when we are quick to jump in to respond, we often spend more time thinking about our response than actively listening to the other person. Be attentive to your voice, your non-verbal behaviours and how they could be interpreted. Keep your intentions central in your mind to avoid entering a right/wrong conversation. Start with understanding the other person first and then seek to be understood.

Further Strategies

Stone et al. (2023) advocate a five-step approach to a meaningful, productive conversation.

1. Prepare by (i) ensuring you understand the facts around the situation; (ii) understanding your emotions within the issue; and (iii) identifying what impact this situation may have on you.
2. Check your intentions and then decide if it is right to raise the issue. What will you accomplish and what is the best way to address the issue?
3. Share your purpose for the conversation and invite the person to resolve the situation, explaining the issue from a third person perspective (as if a neutral person was explaining it). This is similar to partnering language.
4. Explore the other person's story/view and yours. Listen to the other, ask questions and acknowledge feelings. Avoid the right/wrong scenario.
5. Be solution focused and identify options that are mutually beneficial and that keep communication lines open going forward.

Having considered how to have a courageous conversation, we will look at how we can build on these strategies in the context of giving and receiving feedback to colleagues and learners.

GIVING AND RECEIVING FEEDBACK

Feedback in any educational context is important. It helps learners to focus on their future learning and development (feedforward), it helps us evaluate where we are at, and it gives us a degree of objectivity about the context within which we learn, work and interact with others. It can be a useful performance indicator and it informs every human interaction in our professional and personal lives. How we relate to others, build relationships and work collaboratively have all been informed by countless episodes of feedback in different formats across our lives. Indeed, it is often these experiences that shape our value base. Essentially, feedback is a process by which the recipient makes sense of information about their progress or performance and uses it to learn, develop and grow. In this sense, it is driven by the learner or the recipient (Henderson et al. 2019).

When we think about feedback, it is offered, or at least should be offered, to people within the context of agreed values; to share what we value about them, appreciating them to acknowledge their attributes or in appreciating them enough to support their development. Feedback involves sharing what we have observed, and links back to our shared values and our cultures. Person-centred approaches to feedback are founded in honesty, transparency and sincerity, and require us to not just give feedback in a helpful, thoughtful way but also to be open to receiving feedback in order that we can flourish as individuals.

ACTIVITY 5.9

Feedback should be expected but should not be unsolicited or come in a manner that diminishes someone's self-worth. It is important to consider the timing so that a person may be as ready as they can be and prepared to hear it. For feedback to be effective, there needs to be an agreed approach or meeting of minds so that there is reciprocity that leads to personal and professional development. In preparing your approach to feedback, it is important to consider your experience of feedback, when it has helped you to grow and whether it reflected your values. Take some time to consider and respond to the following questions.

What values and principles underpin the feedback I wish to give?

Are those values and principles reflected in my approach to giving feedback?

When you received feedback, what made it beneficial to your development?
What could have been enhanced in the approach used and when is feedback unhelpful?

In view of your experiences, how would you now adapt your approach to feedback?

When is Feedback Criticism and When is it Feedback?

Feedback can be difficult for people to both give and receive. It can be weaponised, insensitive and diminishing if it is not given with the right intention and in the right way. Approaches to giving and receiving feedback should uphold the team's shared values and each individual's personhood. Figure 5.3 sets out some parameters to consider when giving feedback where the intention is to support and empower a person's well-being and development.

Henderson et al. (2019) identified that feedback is successful when there is capacity to engage with feedback, when it is designed correctly and where the culture is right (Table 5.3).

For feedback to be successful, it is important for the recipient to understand what is being shared with them and to be open to considering how they can use this to aid their development. The recipient should adopt a growth mindset and active listening while recognising that how others view us and our performance may differ from our

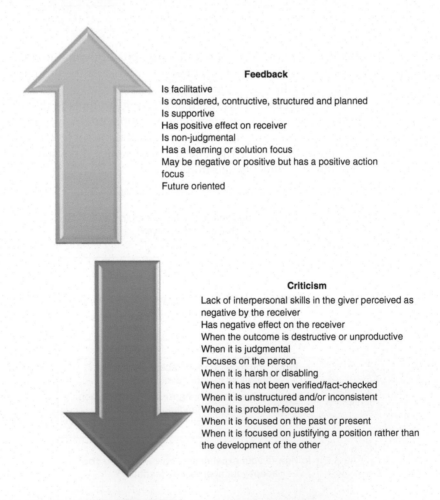

Feedback
Is facilitative
Is considered, contructive, structured and planned
Is supportive
Has positive effect on receiver
Is non-judgmental
Has a learning or solution focus
May be negative or positive but has a positive action focus
Future oriented

Criticism
Lack of interpersonal skills in the giver perceived as negative by the receiver
Has negative effect on the receiver
When the outcome is destructive or unproductive
When it is judgmental
Focuses on the person
When it is harsh or disabling
When it has not been verified/fact-checked
When it is unstructured and/or inconsistent
When it is problem-focused
When it is focused on the past or present
When it is focused on justifying a position rather than the development of the other

FIGURE 5.3 Feedback versus criticism.

TABLE 5.3 Factors for Successful Feedback.

Capacity	Design	Culture
Giver and receiver understand and value feedback	Feedback is provided in a format that the recipient knows how to use	Feedback is a valued and visible enterprise at all levels
The process is an active one for recipients	It is tailored to the recipient	Processes are in place to ensure quality and consistency
Feedback is sought and used to plan and judge effectiveness	The modality of feedback is suited to the circumstance	Feedback is situated in a culture of continuity of vision and commitment
Space and technology facilitate the process of feedback	There is alignment between learning outcomes and multiple tasks	There is flexibility in how to deploy feedback resources to best effect

Source: Adapted from Henderson et al. (2019).

own perspectives. Given that feedback is core to learning and living out shared values, there are some key principles for giving and receiving feedback that we should consider. These are shown in Figure 5.4.

A primary barrier to taking positive action in response to feedback is the recipient's emotional response to the feedback (van der Kleij and Lipnevich 2020; London et al. 2023). The person's response may have been percolating over a period in anticipation of feedback or an emotional response may be triggered based on what is said or not said. Recognising this may be helpful in compassionately acknowledging and reconciling aspects of the emotional response. In so doing, an opportunity may be created to shift the focus of the feedback to capturing its potential for personal learning and development. The person giving the feedback should reflect in and on their approach. They should also be aware of their leadership style and the intended and unforeseen impact of their words or actions on the other person. As a result, the person giving the feedback may need to modify their future approach.

The recipient may seek feedback from more than one person. Triangulating feedback should not be approached with the intention of confirming that personal perspectives are accurate and to invalidate feedback that is not self-satisfying. Instead, using multiple sources of feedback can provide a more comprehensive approach to uncovering personal values and behaviours as the basis for growth as a self-regulating and self-actualising healthcare professional.

EMBEDDING SHARED VALUES

Changes in learning organisations may create the potential for cultural instability or erosion. For example, changes to team membership through natural attrition such as retirements, and the recruitment of new colleagues, may alter the team dynamics.

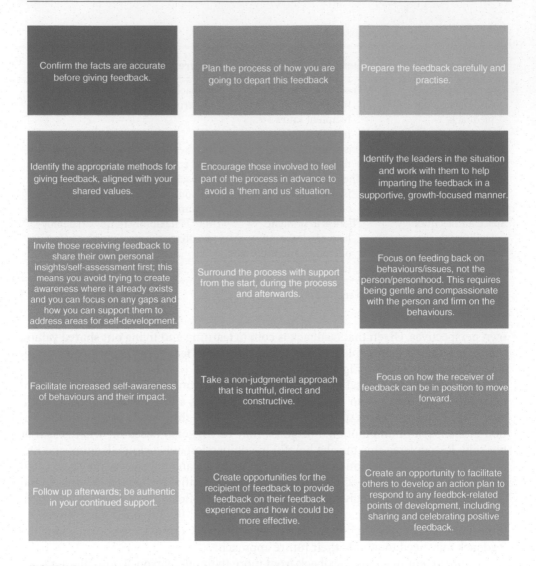

FIGURE 5.4   Principles of giving and receiving feedback.
Source: Adapted from Dewing and Titchen (2007).

These factors may impact the extent to which shared values are known and remain shared. Given that shared values are central to the effectiveness of the complex education system in which curricula operate, culture should be monitored, and strengths, weakness, opportunities and threats explored and managed.

In the next section we will share a case study as an example of how, once a person-centred healthful culture has been established, a team has remained vigilant to monitoring and sustaining it so that it remains alive and healthy. The case study showcases how shared values are the bedrock for the other Ss. In the case study, shared values were used to inform recruitment and selection systems, induction for new colleagues and staff appraisals. Integrating shared values in this way strengthened the infrastructure of the whole system by having a consistent approach where people were supported to actively participate, connect and contribute to person-centred learning cultures.

Case Study 5.1   Embedding Shared Values in a Whole-system Approach to Developing Person-centred Cultures

As discussed earlier in the chapter, McCormack (2022) is explicit that to achieve person-centredness, the culture must be developed and sustained by people who espouse the principles and values of person-centredness. In this section we share some examples about how, once a person-centred healthful culture has been established, a divisional team has worked to keep it alive, growing and sustained through organisational values and systems. This includes approaches to including and supporting new colleagues to move from being present to actively participating, connecting and contributing.

RECRUITMENT AND SELECTION

In recruitment for new staff, job descriptions explicitly state that as a workplace we have person-centred ways of working, shared values and shared decision making. Shortlisted candidates who are invited for interview are asked to bring an artefact with them that they can use to introduce themselves and to explain how their values and beliefs relate to the job they have applied for. Interview questions are competency based but specifically focus on shared values and ways of working. Examples of questions are shown in Table 5.4.

TABLE 5.4   Job-related Competency – Leadership.

Introductory text read to interviewee: We have established a shared governance approach to management and leadership in the Division, meaning all team members contribute to the working of the Division.
1. Can you describe your key qualities as a person and how you bring these to your approach to leadership?
2. Please provide an example of when you have participated in a shared and participatory approach to leadership.
3. What part did you take? How successful was the approach?
4. How did you measure success in this activity?

(continued)

(continued)

SHARED VALUES IN STAFF INDUCTION

On arrival as part of the team, each member of staff is appointed a mentor to meet regularly with them and introduce them to how we as a division fit and collaborate with the wider university while maintaining our own person-centred identity. To

Page | 2

NURSING DIVISION: PERFORMANCE ENHANCEMENT REVIEW (PER) TEMPLATE

Assumptions: Work is engaging and reenergising; Primary aim of work is to flourish; Work adds to the totality of who we are as a person

SECTION 1: FLOURISHING AT WORK This section is to help you record key areas of your job, including a summary of your valued accomplishments to date and share your overall career vision. You may also wish to consider any challenges you have experienced in delivering your objectives.

In my work I am passionate about: *(please complete)*

being in class room with learners

group supervision with learners

explicitly drawing on new research in education

developing my teaching skills

working in this team - most of the time!

My career aspirations are ......*(What do you need to achieve this? How are you going to make this happen?)*

In five years time (approx.) I see myself with a PhD and building a research component to my role. I will probably still be working in this team, if the developments continue.

I know what topic I want to explore and have ideas about what my research would focus on in the longer term

I have to get a PhD or other similar qualification to be a researcher.

I need a better workload balance (less admin) so I can start building up my involvement with research..... I am assuming I can do this before I start a PhD?

I need permission to apply for a doctoral study programme . I am going to fast track my studies and draw on work and publications I have already achieved

I also want some exposure to groups outside of Nursing so I can get more of a sense of what goes on in the school and the university

Version 1 JD Nursing Division May 2019
Adapted from a template devised as part of The National Programme to Enable Person-centred Cultures. HSE Ireland

FIGURE 5.5   Performance enhancement review template.

help in building relationships and orienting new members to the culture and expectations of the team, a series of recorded seminars are facilitated by existing staff covering topics such as 'Person-centred philosophies', 'Divisional shared values', and 'Being a person-centred educator – what does that mean to you?'. The seminars provide a discussion forum and the opportunity for new members of staff to think about the application of person-centred approaches and ways of working in their new workplace. This work is further developed in away days for all staff.

SHARED VALUES IN STAFF APPRAISALS

Annual appraisal or performance enhancement review (Figure 5.5) provides an opportunity for reflection through a person-centred lens to identify what has/has not worked well. During the review, achievements are acknowledged and celebrated. Future goals are identified together with any support needed to help achieve these. There is also the opportunity to think about what being present means and to consider where they feel they are on a continuum from being present to having presence and actively participating, connecting and contributing.

SUMMARY

- In this chapter we have explored why shared values are a prerequisite for establishing and sustaining person-centred learning cultures.
- Making shared values explicit can be achieved by working collaboratively with others to clarify the values that everyone is willing to endorse and live out. When this happens, the shared values will be manifest in the team's behaviours and the culture that is co-created.
- It is important to acknowledge that achieving person-centred learning cultures is a journey rather than a one-off achievement or destination. Embedding shared values requires vision, sustained commitment and collective leadership. When each team member takes ownership and shared responsibility for realising the agreed values, then trust and respect are fostered, partnership working is incentivised and the capacity for transformative change is leveraged.
- Shared values act as a multiplier for a healthful culture. In the case of person-centred cultures, the multiplier effect has the potential to transform not only learning but also the embedding of humanistic approaches into healthcare practice.

REFERENCES

Dewing, J. and Titchen, A. (2007). *Workplace Resources for Practice Development*. London: Royal College of Nursing.

Dewing, J., McCormack, B., and Titchen, A. (2014). *Practice Development Workbook for Nursing, Health and Social Care Teams*. Chichester: Wiley Blackwell.

Drennan, D. (1992). *Transforming Company Culture*. London: McGraw-Hill.

Goddu, A.P., O'Conor, K.J., Lanzkron, S. et al. (2018). Do words matter? Stigmatizing language and the transmission of bias in the medical record. *Journal of General Internal Medicine* 33 (5): 685–691.

Harding, E., Wait, S., and Scrutton, J. (2015). *The State of Play in Person-centred Care: A Pragmatic Review of how Person-centred Care Is Defined, Applied and Measured*. London: Health Policy Partnership.

Henderson, M., Phillips, M., Ryan, T. et al. (2019). Conditions that enable effective feedback. *Higher Education Research and Development* 38 (7): 1401–1416.

Klancnik Gruden, M., Turk, E., McCormack, B., and Štiglic, G. (2021). Impact of person-centred interventions on patient outcomes in acute care settings: a systematic review. *Journal of Nursing Care Quality* 36 (1): E14–E21.

Koenig, S.A. (2013). Courageous conversations. *Nebraska Lawyer* 6: 27–29.

Leplege, A., Gzil, F., Cammelli, M. et al. (2007). Person-centredness: conceptual and historical perspectives. *Disability and Rehabilitation* 29: 20–21.

London, M., Volmer, J., Zyberaj, J., and Kluger, A.N. (2023). Gaining feedback acceptance: leader–member attachment style and psychological safety. *Human Resource Management Review* 33 (2): 100953.

Manley, K., Sanders, K., Cardiff, S., and Webster, J. (2011). Effective workplace culture: the attributes, enabling factors, and consequences of a new concept. *International Practice Development Journal* 1 (2): 1.

Manley, K., O'Keefe, H., Jackson, C. et al. (2014). A shared purpose framework to deliver person-centred, safe and effective care: organisational transformation using practice development methodology. *International Practice Development Journal* 4 (1): 2.

McCormack, B. (2022). Person-centred care and measurement: the more one sees, the better one knows where to look. *Journal of Health Services Research and Policy* 22 (7): 85–87.

McCormack, B. and McCance, T. (2017). *Person-centred Practice in Nursing and Health Care: Theory and Practice*, 2e. Chichester: Wiley Blackwell.

McCormack, B., McCance, T., and Martin, S. (2021). What is person-centredness? In: *Fundamentals of Person-centred Healthcare Practice* (ed. B. McCormack, T. McCance, C. Bulley, et al.), 13–22. Chichester: Wiley Blackwell.

McCormack, B., Magowan, R., O'Donnell, D. et al. (2022). Developing a person-centred curriculum framework: a whole-systems methodology. *International Practice Development Journal* 12 (2): 1–11.

Miles, A. and Asbridge, J.E. (2014). Clarifying the concepts, epistemology and lexicon of person-centeredness: an essential pre-requisite for the effective operationalization of PCH within modern healthcare systems. *European Journal for Person Centered Healthcare* 2 (1): 1–15.

O'Donnell, D. (2021). Learning to Become a Person-Centred Healthcare Professional: A Mixed Methods Study. Doctoral thesis, Ulster University.

O'Donnell, D., Dickson, C., Phelan, A. et al. (2022). A mixed methods approach to the development of a person-centred curriculum framework: surfacing person-centred principles and practices. *International Practice Development Journal* 12 (3): 1–14.

Sanders, K., Webster, J., Manley, K., and Cardiff, S. (2021). Recognising and developing effective workplace cultures across health and social care that are also good places to work. In: *International Practice Development in Health and Social Care*, 2e (ed. K. Manley, V. Wilson, and C. Øye), 205–219. Oxford: Wiley Blackwell.

Stone, D., Patton, B., and Heen, S. (2023). *Difficult Conversations: How to Discuss What Matters Most*. New York: Penguin.

Van der Kleij, F.M. and Lipnevich, A.A. (2020). Student perceptions of assessment feedback: a critical scoping review and call for research. *Educational Assessment, Evaluation and Accountability* 33: 345–373.

Vygotsky, L.S. (1986). *Thought and Language*. Cambridge, MA: MIT Press.

Waterman, J., Peters, T., and Philips, J. (1980). Structure is not organization. *Business Horizons* 23 (3): 14–26.

Wilson, V., Dewing, J., Cardiff, S. et al. (2020). A person-centred observational tool: devising the Workplace Culture Critical Analysis Tool®. *International Practice Development Journal* 10 (1): article 3.

CHAPTER 6

Style

This chapter will explore the meaning of leadership 'style' while leading some aspect of a person-centred curriculum, and how a person-centred approach to leadership can shape the way a programme of work is led. We are aware that leadership can mean different things to different people and that no universally accepted definition exists. However, in this chapter we will be offering activities for individuals and/or teams to engage with and explore the prospect of leading curricula from a person-centred paradigm, thereby achieving congruence between what you aim to achieve and how you go about achieving it.

Alongside exploring the meaning of leadership in the context of a person-centred curriculum, we will invite you to reflect on the extent to which you consider yourself to be a leader (leadership identity), who you are or should be leading (stakeholder engagement), and how you can co-create a culture to achieve the curriculum goals (healthful learning culture) (see Chapters 3 and 8). While there may not be one way to lead a person-centred curriculum, there is sufficient evidence to propose adopting a person-centred approach to leading the development, delivery and evaluation of healthcare curricula. In doing so, you will be contributing to the creation of conditions for human flourishing – the ultimate aim of person-centred practice (see Chapter 8).

INTRODUCTION

This chapter focuses on the leadership 'style' component of the Person-Centred Curriculum Framework. The framework defines a person-centred style of leadership as the 'development, delivery and evaluation of the curriculum as being authentic, collaborative, cooperative and embracing the principles of collective leadership' (Cook et al. 2022, p. 6).

Developing Person-Centred Cultures in Healthcare Education and Practice: An Essential Guide, First Edition.
Edited by Brendan McCormack.
© 2024 John Wiley & Sons Ltd. Published 2024 by John Wiley & Sons Ltd.

In a person-centred curriculum, all stakeholders can engage with the curriculum through democratic and co-creative processes embedded in quality and governance structures and processes. The fostering of trust and utilisation of talents and expertise cultivates a community of person-centred champions who collectively lead the curriculum into the future (Cook et al. 2022) (see also Chapter 8).

Based on educator, regulator and learner perspectives and experiences gathered during the development of the Person-centred Curriculum Framework, five thematic actions were identified for person-centred curriculum leaders. These have guided the information and activities presented in the rest of this chapter.

1. Promoting flexibility, openness, authentic co-operation and democratic processes in the organisation.
2. Creating and supporting an effective community of champions of person-centredness present among all groups involved in curriculum development and delivery (e.g. educators, leaders, managers, students and healthcare practitioners).
3. Fostering recognition, trust and utilisation of member talents and learning needs to ensure action is taken towards developing and delivering a person-centred curriculum/culture.
4. Role modelling person-centred ways of being in actions, presence and authentic involvement, when engaging with others.
5. Using the language of distributed leadership.

WHAT DOES LEADERSHIP MEAN TO YOU?

It could be said that leadership of anything and anyone starts with knowing and leading self. Considering this, we would first like to invite you to explore what you (and other leaders within your curriculum) mean by the term 'leadership'. Also, what happens when you attach the adjectives 'person-centred', 'authentic', 'collaborative' and 'co-operative' to the noun 'leadership'.

ACTIVITY 6.1

OBJECTIVE

This activity helps individuals, groups or teams to develop personal and/or shared understandings of leadership style by exploring how you/your team see leadership and what successful leadership looks like.

MATERIALS NEEDED

Pens, markers, art supplies (e.g. paint, coloured paper, colouring pencils), whiteboard or flipchart.

INSTRUCTIONS

Activities 6.1 and 6.2 can both be undertaken by individuals or a group/team. You will need to complete the first activity in order to develop your understanding of leadership in Activity 6.2. If you are working alone then you may also find it helpful to share your thoughts with another person (e.g. peer, mentor, leader) who can challenge what you are thinking. If you are working as a group/team, you will all need to work together, discuss and come to a shared agreement of what leadership means for you collectively.

1. Introduction (15 minutes)
   If you are completing this activity with a group or team, welcome participants and introduce the activity's objective: to develop personal and shared understandings of leadership style by exploring how the group/team sees leadership and what successful leadership looks like. Explain the steps below one at a time to ensure people are clear about what they are being asked to do.
2. Developing an individual perspective of leadership (15 minutes)
   As an individual, choose or create an object that represents leadership in some way. You may choose an object from your environment, an image from the internet or create an expression using paints, sculpture, a theatre sketch, song or dance.
   - Study the object closely, noting down words of what it 'says' to you in terms of leadership.
3. Developing the imagery to achieve a definition (30 minutes)
   (Individual): Now use the words you applied to the imagery to formulate a short definition of leadership. If you are completing this exercise alone, consider asking a colleague or mentor to help you reflect on your definition, word choice and usage, and so challenge your thinking.
   (Group/team): Invite colleagues to 'read' each other's creative expression too. Discuss and note down on a flipchart agreed words that you all think define leadership. Using these words, formulate your own short definition of leadership. Share it with the group or team and agree an overarching definition.
4. Exploring leadership identity (20 minutes)
   Even if you do not hold a hierarchical leadership/management position within the curriculum, ask yourself: 'According to this definition; (individual) what is my leadership identity and am I (could I be) exercising leadership?' (Group/team) 'What leadership identity do we aspire to and are we (could we be) exercising leadership?'
5. Conclusion (10 minutes)
   Clearly restate the definition. If you are working as an individual, consider sharing your thoughts with a peer or mentor. If you are working as a group/team, and planning to undertake Activity 6.2, summarise the activity, take a short break and explain where and when you will reconvene.

ACTIVITY 6.2

OBJECTIVE

To develop a deeper understanding of leadership style by elaborating your individual or agreed definitions using adjectives.

MATERIALS NEEDED

Internet, access to scholarly articles, pens, markers, creative materials, whiteboard or flipchart.

INSTRUCTIONS

1. Introduction (10 minutes)
   Welcome participants back, if you have had a short break, and outline the objective: to develop a deeper understanding of leadership style by elaborating your individual or agreed definitions using adjectives.
2. Developing deeper understandings (20 minutes)
   Now that you have your individual or team definition of leadership, seek definitions for the following adjectives: authentic/authenticity; collaborative/collaboration; co-operative/co-operation. You may like to search for scholarly articles on authentic, collaborative or co-operative leadership in higher education.
   (Individual) Use the definitions to enhance your short definition of leadership.
   (Group/team) Revisit your definition(s) from Activity 6.1 to compare and contrast your definitions, refining and adapting them until consensus or consent is achieved on a shared understanding.
3. Evaluation and reflection (10 minutes)
   (Individual) Write a reflection on how you found this process and what you have learnt about your leadership style and leadership in general.
   (Group/team) Invite the participants to give you feedback on how they found the process, what they liked best, what they liked least and what they learned about leadership.
4. Conclusion (10 minutes)
   Clearly restate your agreed definition. If you are working with a group/team, summarise the key messages from the activity, agree any actions that need to be taken and who will take the actions.

WHO ARE THE LEADERS?

Although there is no universal contemporary definition of leadership, most definitions include some description of a leader inspiring and motivating others (exerting positive influence) and creating environments (structures, processes and cultures) to achieve (shared) goals. Since the new millennium, there has been a strong movement away from traditional views of leadership being a natural talent or competency only expected of those in hierarchical (management) positions. In collective leadership, all members of a team can potentially lead some aspect of the curriculum based on their capabilities, talents, (learning) needs or experience. This not only respects their right to self-determination, but each person also has space to be the best they can be in what they do, collaborate and actively contribute to realising shared goals. It is a myth that collective leadership negates hierarchical leadership, but hierarchical leaders do need to be responsive – stepping up when a group is not successfully leading itself, stepping back when it is. Given this, you are invited to consider what you could lead, and if you are a hierarchical leader, who could be leading what in the curriculum?

ACTIVITY 6.3

Who is Leading What?

OBJECTIVE

To reflect on and identify your talents, past leadership experiences and learning needs.

MATERIALS NEEDED

Space to reflect individually, notepad/computer.

INSTRUCTIONS

This activity can be undertaken by individual hierarchical leaders to explore their exercising of leadership within the curriculum.

1. Reflection (45 minutes)
   Reflect on and identify your talents, past leadership experiences and learning needs. Some key questions to help are as follows.
   - What have you previously led? Think of workgroups, projects or other activities. What were positive experiences and what were less enjoyable? What made them (less) enjoyable?
   - What do you enjoy doing, and what feels easy and energising in your current role within the curriculum? Is this the same as what others feed back to you? What other skills and qualities do they regularly praise you for?
   - What would you like to develop further/become better at? How could this benefit the design, delivery or evaluation of the curriculum?
   - What would you like to lead within the curriculum? Who needs to know this for it to become reality?
2. Taking action
   To complete this activity, consider who you find it helpful to share your reflective thoughts with (e.g. peer, mentor, leader) who can challenge what you are thinking and to dig deeper.

ACTIVITY 6.4

OBJECTIVE

To enable hierarchical leaders to foster the recognition, trust in and use of team talents when promoting collective leadership.

MATERIALS NEEDED

(Individual) Space to reflect, notepad/computer.
(Group) Room to meet, sticky notes, markers, whiteboard or flipchart, profile cards.

INSTRUCTIONS

This activity can be undertaken by individual hierarchical leaders or group/team members to explore their exercising of leadership within the curriculum. If you are working alone, you may find it helpful to share your thoughts with another person (e.g. peer, mentor, leader) who can challenge what you are thinking and dig deeper. If you are working as a group/team, you can challenge one another.

1. Introduction (10 minutes)
   If you are completing this activity with a group or team, welcome participants and introduce the activity's objective: to foster the recognition, trust in and use of team talents when promoting collective leadership. Explain the steps below one at a time to ensure people are clear about what they are being asked to do.
2. Identifying stakeholders (15 minutes)
   Use index cards (or some other form of documentation) to create 'profiles' of the people you lead/engage with during curriculum design, delivery and evaluation. Start with 9–10 profiles, for instance: (i) five people who are engaged daily in the curriculum, three of whom you know well and two you know less well; (ii) three people who are regularly engaged in the curriculum, one you know well and two you know a little; (iii) one person you do not know well and is occasionally engaged in the curriculum.
3. Identifying team talents (20 minutes)
   For each person, identify:
   - their role in the curriculum: are they an educator (lecturer, preceptor, etc.)/ supporter (administrative, advisory, etc.)/learner (student council, interest group, etc.)/regulator (internal or external)?
   - their talents/strengths – what are they good at (in your experience/you hear others acknowledge)?
   - the areas of engagement: where/what are they currently active in?
   - the level(s) of engagement – are they highly engaged; intermittently engaged; occasionally engaged; unknown?
   - their potential value – where could their talents be best/better suited?
   - their needs – what would they like to be (more) engaged in?

4. Formulating the team
(Individual) Plan short 'coffee' conversations with each person to: (i) verify your assumptions; (ii) explore potentials; (iii) plan actions.
(Group/team) Decide which member of the group/team will have a short coffee conversation with each identified person (this should be a shared activity between all the team). Plan a meeting date to come back together to discuss the outcome of your conversations and plan the next action (30 minutes).
Repeat steps 2–4, thereby expanding your scope of stakeholders and their (potential) engagement.

LEADING IN A PERSON-CENTRED WAY

One definition of leadership could be 'the unifying of people to collectively achieve a shared purpose'. As such, this could be applied to any context, from leading the care of one patient (micro-level), to leading a Bachelor program on physiotherapy (meso-level), to leading an (inter)national community of practice for person-centred healthcare (macro-level). The definition denotes a process of initiating and maintaining relationships, whereby leadership now becomes a relational practice: something that is exercised, developed and manifest in relationships.

Defining leadership as a relational practice helps align it to 'person-centred practice'. Janssen and Jacobs (2018) define person-centred practice as the continuous process of collectively forming relationships and structures within care, learning and working environments, whereby self-determination and dignity of all are realised. In the context of healthcare curricula, this can include educator–student (learning) relationships as well as educator–educator or student–student (collegial) and leadership relationships. Fundamentally, person-centredness centralises personhood and is about forming healthful relationships characterised by mutual respect and understanding for who we are, and a person's right to self-determination (McCormack and McCance 2017).

Our theoretical understanding of person-centredness has emerged through research focusing on collaborative approaches to improving practice that keeps persons central to changes being made (e.g. Manley et al. 2011; Cardiff et al. 2020). These researchers have recommended a leadership style that is transformational. An example is Kouzes and Posner's (2017) framework of five practices for exemplary leadership: modelling the way; inspiring a shared vision; encouraging the heart; enabling others to act; and challenging the process. More recently, person-centred approaches to leadership have been inductively developed within healthcare contexts (Cummings et al. 2018; Lynch et al. 2017). While we would highly recommend reading all these resources for depth and clarity, we have synthesised some key messages emerging from that body of work and in so doing articulate a description for person-centred healthcare curricula.

- Leaders of person-centred healthcare curricula intentionally foster healthful work and learning environments where all can come into their own and flourish. In doing so, stakeholders collaboratively, co-operatively and collectively design, deliver and evaluate educational programmes for the development of future person-centred healthcare professionals.

■ Being present and connected – authentically caring and other-centred leaders who are present in the moment and situations can build relational connectedness with and among those involved in the curriculum. They use all their senses to gather information about those they are leading, interpreting this against a backdrop of individual, group and organisational particularities (social, historical and environmental contexts). Their presence is felt, even during their physical absence, as stakeholders actively and collectively work towards a shared vision without jeopardising individual needs.

■ Harmonising and aligning visions – person-centred leaders inspire the identification and embodiment of shared values and beliefs, individually and collectively, through communing (action-orientated dialogue) in critical and creative learning spaces.

■ Balancing needs – working towards the enactment of a shared vision, leaders are constantly questioning the status quo as they endeavour to balance the needs of individuals with those of self and others, all within existent (internal and external) regulations. Systematic and systemic evaluation aids the process of gaining insight into (the balancing of) needs.

■ Enabling movement – reflexive leaders who listen with the heart are continuously responsive, constantly repositioning themselves in relation to the other person to motivate continued action, growth and development.

VISIONING LEADERSHIP FOR A PERSON-CENTRED CURRICULUM

Being able to articulate your own individual or collective definition of effective leadership can be challenging, especially if you do not know how to structure it or think that it needs to be done all at once and for all time. By definition, visions are descriptions of an idealised state that represent the values, assumptions and information (contextual, propositional, experiential knowledge) that exist at the time the vision is formed (see Chapter 2). All these values, ideas and knowledge evolve with time. Because of this, visions should be revisited frequently for improvement, whether they be personal visions or collective visions on how to lead a person-centred curriculum.

Walker and Avant's (2011) basic framework for a concept is a useful tool for constructing a personal/collective vision for person-centred leadership in a person-centred curriculum. If you have completed the earlier exercises in this chapter, you will have made a start on determining the content of the framework, although they were not focused on a person-centred approach to leadership.

ACTIVITY 6.5

OBJECTIVE

To analyse the concept of leading a person-centred curriculum.

MATERIALS NEEDED

Whiteboard, flipchart, sticky notes, art supplies (paints, coloured pencils, markers), the conceptual framework in Figure 6.1.

INSTRUCTIONS

1. Introduction (10 minutes)
   Welcome participants and introduce the activity's objective: to analyse the concept of leading a person-centred curriculum.
2. Creating a creative expression (15 minutes)
   Invite participants to choose or create a creative expression of what person-centred leadership would look like when leading a curriculum. Do not spend much time 'thinking' about the creative expression, let your eyes and hands move freely and follow your instinct.
3. Developing key words (20 minutes)
   Study your own (and other people's) creative expression, identifying key words and phrases it/they evoke in you, particularly words and phrases you associate with person-centredness. Write these down on sticky notes and place them on the expression(s) at appropriate points.
4. Achieving consensus (40 minutes)
   Collect the post-its and cluster those of identical/similar meaning. Allocate them to the various sections within the concept analysis framework (see Figure 6.1). Some rewording/rephrasing may be needed for them to 'fit' the section.

   When working towards a collective vision, ensure that consensus or consent is explicitly achieved for each allocation. The following questions may help the process.
   - Does this describe a leader trait/characteristic consistent with being a person-centred leader?
   - Does this describe a leadership process, what the leader does to lead those involved in curriculum design, delivery and evaluation?

Short personal definition of good curriculum leadership		
Antecedents and influencing factors	Essential prerequisites	Outcomes
	Characteristics:	
	Practices:	

FIGURE 6.1   A concept analysis framework of leadership in a person-centred curriculum.

(continued)

(continued)

- Does this describe an influencing factor, that which enables or hinders leader being and doing?
- Does this describe the outcome, consequence or result of the leadership enacted by the leader?

5. Achieving a collective vision (30 minutes)

   Contemplate the 'essence' of leading a person-centred curriculum and use the concept analysis framework content to formulate a concise yet meaningful definition. When working towards a collective vision, ensure that consensus or consent is explicitly achieved for the final statement.

6. Conclusion (10 minutes)

   Conclude by summarising your collective definition and vision. Ask for feedback to evaluate the process and how you led this activity.

NAVIGATING TENSIONS, DANCING WITH PERSONS

As the concept analysis framework shows, while a leader's intended performance may be based on their individual vision of leadership, leadership practice is also contextualised, influenced by surrounding persons, events, structures and processes. Leading by being in relation with others and embedded in contexts is fraught with tensions as neither persons nor contexts are stable entities. As such, leadership is sometimes compared to improvised dance as the leader navigates influencing factors while trying to respond appropriately to their dance partner. It requires a large amount of self- and contextual awareness, as well as using emotional and interpersonal intelligences to learn and adapt (this is explored further in section 'Knowing self as an emotionally intelligent and resonant leader'). Figure 6.2 outlines some tensions commonly experienced by leaders (Jordan et al. 2020) and offers questions for you to consider.

Working from the same assumption that navigating tensions while dancing with others is a continuous process, Cardiff et al. (2018) (describe four basic leader stances/positions. They also emphasis that there is no fixed pattern to using the stances. Leader stance will constantly change as the leader responds to changes within the person(s) they are leading and contextual dynamics.

- Leading from the front = offering to 'show' how to move forward.
- Leading from the side-line = offering 'instructions' for moving forward.
- Leading from alongside = using high challenge in combination with high support to enable movement.
- Leading from behind = stepping back, creating space and observing how the other person(s) moves.

To lead in a person-centred way, it is useful to become aware of which stances you tend to take as a leader, in different situations and with different people, while navigating tensions. Reflecting on tensions and leadership stances will enhance your ability to be flexible and take appropriate action.

- Expert v Learner: Leaders may be experts, but no leader is an expert in everything. Consequently, as a leader you should know when to be a learner too.

  • What expertise do you bring to the curriculum? What areas do you need to/want to learn more about? Are you aware of who has the expertise needed?

- Constant v Adaptor: Having a clear (shared) vision and keeping to it in times of uncertainty can be reassuring and motivational for others, but being too rigid and unable to adapt to change can be detrimental.

  • How clear is your vision, and how do you know that stakeholders still understand where you want to go with the curriculum? (see Chapter 2).

- Tactician v Visionary: Whilst being able to clearly articulate an ambitious vision of where you want to work towards with the curriculum, it also needs to be grounded and realistic.

  • How do stakeholder claims and concerns fit with the feasibility of your vision? Do you need to refine or affirm your vision?

- Teller v Listener: Clearly articulating where you want to move towards with the curriculum is important for inspiring and motivating others, but no leader is an expert in all areas influencing the feasibility of a curriculum strategy.

  • What opposing and complimentary views have you heard (recently)? When and where do you need to listen next before making (shared) decisions?

- Power-over v Power-with: A leader position usually brings with it power. Power can be viewed neutrally as the possibility of making decisions and taking action to achieve a desired outcome. This can be exerted by an individual or group whereby the outcomes will affect others, but they have not been included in the decision-making process. There may be times when this is unavoidable or even welcomed by those others. Power can also be exerted with others (power-with) whereby those affected by the outcomes of the decisions and actions are co-deciders and co-actors.

  • When did you last exert 'power-over' others? When did you last exert 'power-with' others? Who were involved, who not? Under what circumstances were the decisions made? What were the consequences? For whom? Were the right decisions made? For whom?

- Intuition v Analytics: Making decisions can be a reactionary or contemplated response. The basis upon which we make decisions is related to the time and information available. A danger is relying solely upon one source of knowledge. Whilst intuitive responses can be valid and helpful, a failure to incorporate analytics could reduce effectiveness or efficiency. The evidence-based movement in healthcare has taught us that ideally we should base decisions on a blending of knowledge from various sources: propositional, experiential and contextual.

  • What is your tendency: intuitive or analytical leadership? What sources of knowledge could you better utilise? Who are experts in this field who could assist you and your team?

- Perfectionism v Acceleration: Whilst there may be a desire to craft the perfect curriculum, the ideal as described by all stakeholders may be unachievable. Remaining in the design modus may also backfire in terms of working towards the curriculum strategy. As a leader you will be constantly charged with monitoring design and development activities in light of an evolving context.

  • What in your curriculum design and development can be further perfected before being launched? What needs to be accelerated before it becomes 'too little too late'?

FIGURE 6.2 Tensions experienced by leaders.

ACTIVITY 6.6

OBJECTIVE

To reflect on different stances.

MATERIALS NEEDED

Space to reflect, notepad/computer/reflective diary or scrapbook. This will enable you to make creative images.

INSTRUCTIONS

Think of a situation or tension and write it down as concretely as you can.

1. What was the tension about and what are the characteristics of the tension?
2. Who were involved and which roles did the persons in the tension have?
3. What is your role?
4. What are your feelings?
5. Which stance did you take and what made you take that stance?
6. How did it work out?
7. What could/would you do different next time?

KNOWING SELF AS A LEADER

Throughout this chapter, we have emphasised the importance of knowing self in order to be an effective leader. In a person-centred world, knowing self as an individual is defined as the way a person makes sense of their knowing, being and becoming (Brown and Tropea 2021). Knowing self is important, as it is our relationship with self that forms the foundation from which our relationships with others are built (Lynch et al. 2021). Self is not a fixed entity, and it too changes in different situations and over time. Philosophers, psychologists and sociologists all have proposed different theories and definitions of self (see Stevens 2002 or Zahavi 2014 to explore what resonates with you). When taken in isolation, often these perspectives provide a fragmented view of self. However, in person-centredness, the components of self encompass biological, psychological, social, environmental and spiritual elements and the four dimensions of being a person (McCormack and McCance 2017).

ACTIVITY 6.7

OBJECTIVE

To develop your understanding and apply the components of knowing self.

MATERIALS NEEDED

Computer, notepad, reflective diary or scrapbook.

INSTRUCTIONS

Read the following scenario and then answer these questions.

- Can you think of other examples of each of the components of self?
- What are the leader's 'hot buttons': things that trigger a strong or negative emotional response (Masterson 2007)?

  Do different situations make you react in different ways? What are your 'hot buttons'?

SCENARIO

Chloé has been asked to lead a small group of educators and students to develop an undergraduate module focusing on person-centred leadership. Having never led this type of activity before, Chloé is apprehensive, questioning if she can do this. Knowing self, she accepts that she is conscientious and prone to anxiety (biological). However, she is highly motivated and resilient which helps her to focus on the task in hand (psychological). Chloé is well educated and has a good home support system (social), which enables her to feel a sense of belonging and to connect with others easily (spiritual). Being aware of her person-centred values, she knows that she does not function at her best when working in an environment where people do not listen to alternative views, respect one another or have a willingness to reach consensus. For this reason, Chloé realises that to successfully lead the group, she will be required to clearly communicate the purpose of the group, co-create principles for working together and ensure that she facilitates discussions, using high challenge/high support, to create a psychologically safe environment in which all can engage in the process to achieve an outcome (environmental). She also appreciates that reflecting on her leadership will help her to grow as a person and leader.

Accepting that the world is not constant and that we are not static beings, it stands to reason that the road to understanding and knowing self has the propensity to change over time (Brown and Tropea 2021). We learn about self every day in relation with others and constantly alter our perspectives (Van Lieshout 2017). Therefore, knowing self is not solely focused on the individual – it also acknowledges the connectivity we have with others. This is explored more fully below in knowing self as an emotionally intelligent and resonant leader.

To develop leadership strategies that encourage independent and deliberate reflection on how external challenges may affect the internal self requires bravery and living with uncertainty (Bolton 2014). Standing back to examine what we are doing and the assumptions we make (reflexivity) raises awareness of the influences that surround us and can motivate change (Seedhouse 2017). Thus, finding ways to enhance our self-awareness is essential to leading and delivering a person-centred curriculum.

The person-centred leadership literature describes a leader who is both reflective and reflexive. Where reflection entails reviewing encounters in order to try and understand the world around us, reflexivity is more introspective as we also consider how our own values, beliefs, thought processes and virtues influence how we relate with others and the world around us (Bolton and Delderfield 2018). There are many reflection and reflexive tools and methods available. Unfortunately, some may not feel practical for a busy working environment and reflection/reflexivity is often rushed or occurs more in the preconscious mind than the conscious one. The example tools below offer a compact structure which can be used to reflect on your leadership, depending on whether you move from a reflective mode to a reflexive mode during the process.

Tools to Learn About Self

These tools can be used either as an individual experience or shared with others to enable critical reflection on our own actions. By becoming aware of why we act in certain ways, we can be open to the potential for learning and change.

Journalling – as an individual you may wish to keep a journal to record your thoughts, feelings, experiences and learning with the explicit intention of focusing on understanding self and increasing your self-awareness as you lead curriculum development, delivery and evaluation. There are many mediums open to you to achieve this (a written journal, computer-based journal or creating a picture). Regardless of method, you will perhaps wish to consider:

- what form it will take (e.g. written, electronic, creative)
- how much time you will have to dedicate to your journal
- is it a private journal or one to be shared – for example, with a group of like-minded peers?

For creative journalling ideas, you may wish to access: www.pcp-icop.org. There are also a variety of apps available so that you can write at any time (e.g. reflectly.app; longwalks.com).

Critical ally/friend/companionship (see Chapter 8) – in these approaches to person-centred learning, two colleagues accompany one another on a facilitative, supportive, experiential learning journey. One person is an experienced mentor/facilitator who enables the other person to develop new knowledge and ways of knowing, over time (Titchen et al. 2013; Hardiman and Dewing 2014). This way of understanding self requires working with a defined set of principles to ensure that a psychologically safe space is created for meaningful learning to occur (Brown and McCormack 2016). For further information please see: www.fons.org/Resources.

Learning sets – these offer a more structured approach to learn more about self in the company of others. You could organise a learning set of 6–8 people who are working in higher education and/or practice settings and who want to learn together about

TABLE 6.1 Setting Principles For Working Together.

Learning set
Under each heading, draw out what *behaviours* your group should display for you all to work together safely and in a person-centred way.
Working principles:
- Being compassionate
- Being courageous
- Being open and honest
- Being present
- Being accountable

creating, delivering and evaluating a person-centred curriculum based on one another's experiences. This is a valuable way to learn about leadership with a group of people for a set period of time. Learning sets are usually action orientated with a professional development focus and work on the notion of creating a psychologically safe space. The 'set' normally has a facilitator who is also part of the group and has responsibility for creating the conditions for learning. Prior to commencing working together, principles and behaviours for working are agreed amongst the group, written down and used to ensure a safe environment of high challenge/high support (see principles in Table 6.1). During the sessions, each member is allocated a time slot to discuss their issues while the other group members encourage reflectivity and reflexivity by asking open-ended questions. If you wish to explore this further, you are invited to access: https://rapidbi. com/action-learning-action-learning-sets reg-revens.

Knowing Self as an Emotionally Intelligent and Resonant Leader

Simply knowing and understanding self is not enough to become an effective person-centred leader. Person-centredness is founded on authentic, respectful relationships that honour personhood and lead to the development of mutual trust and understanding. This requires leaders to be aware of, understand and master their own emotions, recognise the emotions of others and manage them depending on each situation (Emotional Intelligence [EI]; Goleman 1995). Research suggests that EI is developmental in nature, with people being able to enhance their emotional skills over time (Wang et al. 2011). Leaders who know themselves well and develop their EI skills become more capable of being flexible, adapting to change and collaborating openly with their team, as they learn how and when to adopt different leadership styles depending on the presenting circumstances. Having undertaken research exploring situational leadership and its links to person-centredness, Lynch et al. (2021) contend that knowing and understanding self from an emotionally intelligent perspective enables leaders to consistently be there for others while also caring for themselves.

This links EI closely to resonant leadership which offers a relationally focused leadership style associated with a commitment to personal values, creating conditions for people to achieve their best, promoting engagement with others and developing positive workplace environments (Cummings et al. 2014). Goleman et al. (2013) propose that leaders' emotions resemble sound waves that resonate with others and positively impact on the emotional climate of a team. When a self-aware, empathetic leader uses excellent communication skills to set a clear purpose and inspire others to embrace activities to achieve group outcomes, colleagues are guided onto a positive wavelength. Such leaders convert challenges to opportunities to create and inspire positive and vibrant workplace environments (Goleman et al. 2013).

The four resonant leader types are as follows.

1. Visionary – inspiring their team, setting a sense of direction, giving feedback in a natural way and providing a clear picture of the future.
2. Coaching – as they show genuine interest in the goals, challenges and personal development of individuals. They individualise assignments to support and develop people.
3. Affiliative – by seeking group harmony, building emotional and social capital, they create positive and supportive cultures.
4. Democratic – through encouraging participation of all team members, valuing the input of others and listening to feedback, consensus is reached and co-operation is enhanced.

Each of these leadership types offers a way to work with students, individuals and teams to create positive learning environments and complement person-centred ideals. It stands to reason that leaders who do not demonstrate skills of emotional intelligence and/or resonant leadership qualities are more likely to create cultures of dissonance and not achieve a harmonious outcome.

ACTIVITY 6.8

OBJECTIVE

To reflect on self as you work towards being a resonant person-centred leader.

MATERIALS NEEDED

Computer, notepad, reflective diary or scrapbook.

INSTRUCTIONS

1. Reflect on the questions below, taken from the Management Support Scale (Cummings et al. 2018). You may wish to complete these questions from two different perspectives: (i) as a person being led by someone else; (ii) as a leader leading others.

   For the first perspective, simply answer the questions as formulated below, with the 'supervisor' being the person leading you. For the second perspective, replace the term supervisor with self (e.g. I treat people with respect, I treat people fairly). You can use a four-point Likert scale to answer each item: often, sometimes, rarely, never.

- My supervisor treats me with respect.
- My supervisor treats me fairly.
- My supervisor shows a genuine interest in me as a person, not just as an employee.
- My supervisor encourages and supports my professional development.
- I am comfortable discussing work-related concerns and issues with my supervisor.
- My supervisor gives me credit and recognition when I do a good job.
- My supervisor gives me feedback that helps me improve my performance.
- My supervisor encourages me to suggest improvements at work.
- My supervisor informs and guides me.
- I feel supported in my work.
- Generally speaking, I am satisfied with my supervisor.

2. Having answered the questions:

What do the answers tell you about 'self': how you experience the leadership of others, and how you yourself practise leadership? What do you value?

What might you want to develop further to become more of a resonant leader?

Knowing self, being emotionally intelligent and developing resonant leadership skills help us to authentically engage with individuals and teams to create psychologically safe spaces as we demonstrate concern for others, listen to opinions, recognise poor behaviours, adjust our emotional responses and challenge people appropriately. This enables person-centred leaders who are developing self to focus on demonstrating their beliefs and values by 'modelling the way' in their interactions with learners, colleagues and key stakeholders (Kouzes and Posner 2017). In our daily interactions, we can role model our values by shaping our observations and evaluations of what is going on.

ACTIVITY 6.9

OBJECTIVE

To develop reflective and reflexive leadership skills.

MATERIALS NEEDED

A reflective diary or scrapbook is recommended.

(continued)

(continued)

INSTRUCTIONS

When resources, particularly time and energy, are limited there is a tendency for us to be more of a spectator (outsider) than participant (insider) when reviewing events. Lengthy tools and methods are therefore not conducive to inspiring reflective leadership practice.

1. Developing a reflection habit (15 minutes/week)
   In your diary, allocate 15 minutes per week to systematically and consistently reflect on your leadership, aided by the questions below.
       Find a quiet space where you will not be disturbed. Recollect an event that made an impact on you (whether that be positive or negative) this week.
   - What was I leading?
   - Who was I leading?
   - Where did I want to lead them towards?
   - Why me and why there?
   - What was the consequence of my leadership?
   - What influenced how I led?
   - To what extent was I leading in a person-centred way?
   - How should I lead such a situation? What stances would be preferable at what moments?
2. Revisiting your reflections
   Once recorded, their meaning will return when you revisit the book. If time permits, spend longer on each question or return to one or more questions after initially working through all seven.

PSYCHOLOGICAL SAFETY AND LEADERSHIP

Working through the previous exercises, you may have appreciated the importance of feeling safe. As a person-centred leader, you will also feel a responsibility to (co-)create psychologically safe environments.

The concept of psychological safety (see Chapter 5) is based on the notion that environmental conditions are created to allow people to safely express their thoughts and ideas without feeling a threat of loss of self-identity or integrity (Schein 2010). Particularly in highly uncertain and dynamic environments, there is a need for leaders to support people to contribute to the conversation, share their view and feel valued. Ultimately, this is essential to organisational learning (Edmondson 2012) as person-centred leaders create critical and creative communicative/learning environments (Cardiff et al. 2018). To help you to create the conditions for a psychological safe space there are six simple steps.

1. Create an environment of openness – principles for working that everyone contributes to making and signs up to.

2. Frame the work as a learning problem – make explicit that there is uncertainty ahead and we need all people to work together to bring their full selves.
3. Acknowledge own fallibility – e.g. I may miss something, and I need your views/thoughts/ideas.
4. Model curiosity – ask lots of questions and actively listen to the responses.
5. Take action – if you agree an action, implement, test, evaluate and review it.
6. Reflect – on what you have achieved, and what needs to be amended.

When leading a person-centred curriculum, we need to find ways to work effectively across academic and practice settings. We also need to build healthful cultures where the needs of self and others are considered, ensuring everyone has an equal voice, as well as their contribution being valued and respected (Edmondson 2012). Without this, learners, other key stakeholders and people who use health services may become uninterested in contributing to developing curricula. So, reflexive person-centred leaders should consider how they can create psychologically safe environments to enable stakeholders to co-create, deliver and evaluate curricula.

ACTIVITY 6.10

OBJECTIVE

To reflect on strategies to enhance your leadership style.

MATERIALS NEEDED

Computer, notepad, reflective diary or scrapbook.

INSTRUCTIONS

Read and reflect on the scenarios presented below, or similar situations you have experienced.

- Consider the reactions. What values were being demonstrated?
- Why was the situation (not) psychologically safe? What else could have been done?

SCENARIO 1

A programme leader observed a student being prevented from sharing their thoughts during a training session. This was raised as a concern with the trainee educator. To create a psychologically safe space, without blame, the programme lead invited the trainee to talk about which students were included in the discussion. Having completed feeding back and discussing observations made, the programme lead suggested they collaboratively think about what they can do with the conclusions they

(continued)

(continued)

had drawn about the different ways educators can respond to student participation, and in particular those they felt were in keeping with person-centred values.

SCENARIO 2

A team leader became aware of a situation where, through the standardised central university evaluation system, students were inappropriately criticising named individuals of the teaching team. This system was designed to send unedited comments directly to the team involved, which was now causing significant hurt and upset among the teaching team. The team requested a meeting to discuss what had happened and to try to find a way of avoiding a repeat scenario. Previous system hiccups had not been dealt with well and the team leader found that a divergence and avoidance strategy worked best for them. The leader sent a memo explaining that IT had been contacted and they were working on a solution. In addition, the leader decided to speak personally with those affected, thinking it inappropriate to organise a separate meeting, especially considering the current complaints within the team about heavy workloads.

DEVELOPING A STRONG LEADERSHIP IDENTITY

Undoubtedly, you will have noted that having a clear vision on good leadership and knowing self will not guarantee that your (leadership) actions will result in a desired effect. Contextual influences such as the social role you fulfil, the moment in time, the space you inhabit, as well as other internal and external factors, will impact on whether or not you take on a leader role/position. The decision may sometimes be conscious, sometimes not. Working with knowledge on how context is influencing your leadership stance (Van Lieshout 2013), whether to lead or not, and to what extent, is a demonstration of strong leadership identity (Coninck et al. 2023). Strong leadership identity helps people stand firm while remaining responsive to what is needed in the presenting situation and context. It creates a firm basis for enacting self-determination and making deliberate choices that do justice to yourself and others within that situation. Enhancing 'muchness' (Sanders 2021) and enabling self and others to come into their own (Cardiff et al. 2018) is characteristic of person-centred leadership and healthful cultures.

Developing healthful cultures for a person-centred curriculum is known to be complex and dynamic, sown with a variety of tensions for leaders to deal with and decision to be made (Jordan et al. 2020). A willingness to show one's own vulnerability in terms of 'I can' or 'I cannot (at the moment)', and awareness of how you want to be recognised and approached as a leader, are signs of strength, not weakness. They reveal your personhood and when achieved collectively, encourage diversity and appropriate skill mix within a team (see Chapter 8). Reflexive actions enable the continuous updating of the personal 'i-cloud' of characteristics and qualities which can be utilised appropriately.

Leadership identity becomes a navigation panel for being and becoming a leader, and the engine to enacting your (personal) vision of good leadership.

Developing your leadership identity entails answering the question: 'Who is the leader I want to be?' It helps to critically draw on the rich source of available theories and views about leadership. Reflecting on the questions in Activity 6.11 (dialogue with self) as well as engaging in a critical dialogue with an ally, friend or companion will aid clarity, depth and deliberate intention to take position. Remember, this activity is not restricted to those leaders in hierarchical leadership positions. Anyone can be a leader of something, they just need to be(come) aware of their leadership identity.

ACTIVITY 6.11

OBJECTIVE

To sketch out your leadership identity through reflection.

MATERIALS NEEDED

Computer, notepad, reflective diary or scrapbook.

INSTRUCTIONS

1. Think about all you have learnt in this chapter to reflect on the following questions.
   - What images and assumptions about leadership have I been raised with?
   - What is important to me when working with others?
   - What am I prepared/do I feel comfortable to take responsibility for?
   - How do I see my role in the group and the realisation of our mission?
   - When am I allowed (by myself or others) to be a 'boss'?
2. Reflect now on leadership within your team.
   - How do we lead a person-centred curriculum in the right direction?
   - How do we utilise leadership within the group?
   - What influence does organisational structure have on the diverse leadership identities within the group?
   - What leadership vision does the organisation propagate?
   - What strategies could further help the leadership 'fingerprints' of individuals and the team?

Every human being possesses virtues or, rather, shows virtuous behaviour. Virtues are part of one's professional identity. Think of caring or having a sense of responsibility, reliability, curiosity. Moore (2017, p. 115) describes a set of virtues that belong specifically to leaders: integrity, justice, honesty, courage, temperance, practical wisdom, having confidence and being trustworthy and generous. The leadership virtue *par excellence* is the ability to find the right middle ground where you can balance, on the one hand, the virtues consistent with yourself and, on the other hand, the reality around you (the different interests of people and groups). Aristotle called this ability justice, which links strongly with values underlying person-centredness.

Perhaps there are virtues that you think you possess but that have not yet really become characteristics of your being or that you have yet to really internalise. Virtues can be developed and you can become better at them through practice and reflection. By entering transactions with fellow human beings, you can achieve a certain degree of excellence in becoming and being a more virtuous self.

ACTIVITY 6.12

Download the Virtues App on Google Play
Make a selection of what virtues you and/or your team think are important.
Discuss which need further development and how you can achieve that and what support is needed.

LEADING OTHERS TO CREATE HEALTHFUL CULTURES

The intention of a person-centred curriculum is to achieve a healthful learning culture regardless of what is being taught/studied. We have come to realise that how healthcare professionals are educated within the educational and healthcare organisations is fundamental to the type of learning culture created. In this section we consider what these healthful learning cultures look like and how they contribute to human flourishing.

Previously in this chapter, you have had the opportunity to reflect on how you intend to lead a person-centred curriculum. Now we move on to consider how you would know if you had been successful in fostering healthful learning cultures. The activities below are again visualisation exercises but with a different focus: a healthful learning culture. You are also encouraged to again include various key elements of the Person-centred Curriculum Framework in your reflections.

ACTIVITY 6.13

OBJECTIVE

This exercise is designed to help identify these influencing aspects of culture.

MATERIALS NEEDED

Pen(s) and some paper or art materials. Ask the group to have paper and pens ready to reflect after the visualisation. A place/room to sit (or lie down) somewhere quiet, where you will not be disturbed and you are comfortable.

INSTRUCTIONS

Having spent considerable time looking at your self, we now encourage you to think of the departmental and organisational processes that support or hinder your chosen approach to leadership. The activity needs to be at least 30–40 minutes if it is to be beneficial. For this activity you will need the following.

1. A facilitator script to guide an eight-minute visualisation exercise
   'If you are sitting comfortably ... Close your eyes, or allow your gaze to soften and fall beyond the end of your nose. Imagine you are standing outside your workplace. Take a moment. Be still. Notice your surroundings. What do you see, what do you hear? How are you feeling? In your hand you have an invisible cloak. Put it on ... one arm in, your other arm in. Pull your cloak around you and feel yourself dissolve out of sight. The tip of your head is disappearing, your face and neck. Your body, arms, your legs and feet. You are now completely invisible. Take a deep breath in. Let it go. Take another breath in and go through the doors. As you move inside your workplace, people ignore you as they cannot see or hear you. You can see and hear them. Move around freely, noticing who is there, what they are doing and how they are doing it. What are they saying and how are they saying it? What else can you see? Can you smell anything? What else can you hear? Now feel yourself rise and circle above your workplace. The view is different. When you have seen and heard enough, return to the ground and the doors leading outside. When you are ready, take a deep breath in and on the exhale, take your invisible cloak off and feel yourself reappearing. First the top of your head, your face and neck. Your body, your arms, then your legs and feet ... In silence, spend 15 minutes reflecting on what you saw. Document it in writing/a doodle/a mindmap/or a creative expression.'
2. Group discussion (20 minutes)
   Use the following questions.
   - What impact did the physical environment have on the way things were being done?
   - Who did you see and what skill-mix was evident?
   - What did you hear and what did it say about how staff relate to each other?
   - What did leadership look like?
   - How were decisions being made?
   - Where did power mechanisms manifest and what was their influence on the way things were done?
   - How were organisational systems helping or hindering the team to educate learners in a person-centred manner?
3. Conclusion (10 minutes)
   Conclude by summarising your discussion. Ask for feedback to evaluate the process and how this activity was led.

The visualisation exercise should foster insight into the various relationships within the workplace, the systems and the processes. In terms of the leadership relationships, according to the Person-centred Curriculum Framework, leaders of a person-centred curriculum will:

- embrace partnership working for the shared purpose of humanising healthcare
- engage in authentic, collaborative, co-operative processes that embrace the principles of 'collective leadership' in co-creative processes
- apply collective leadership principles to quality and governance structures and processes
- facilitate collective leadership for delivering curriculum outcomes.

These outcomes are features of what McCormack and McCance (2017) refer to as healthful cultures and give us signposts to what we need to pay attention to. A well-known definition of culture is 'the way things are done around here' (Drennan 1992, p. 3) but in reality, culture is much more complex than that. Factors within the curriculum environment can enable or hinder the creation of healthful cultures and it is worth taking time to understand what these are. McCormack and McCance suggest a healthful culture is:

> ... one in which decision making is shared, staff relationships are collaborative, leadership is transformational, innovative practices are supported and is the ultimate outcome for teams working to develop a workplace that is person centred (McCormack and McCance 2017, p. 60).

Relationships are key to embedding the Person-centred Curriculum Framework and from a person-centred perspective, relationships have the intention of mutual learning and growth. Mackay et al. (2021) describe such relationships as healthful relationships in their work with clinical supervisors and students in practice. They suggest that healthful relationships are evident when persons experience a 'sense of being in practice together while supporting each other to seek their full potential' (Mackay and Jans 2022, p. 232). The authors go on to describe relationships that are mutually respectful, accepting of differences, have shared expectations, offer hope and are open to learning, unlearning and relearning.

Healthful relationships are hallmarks of healthful cultures and leadership is of course a catalyst for creating such cultures. Cardiff et al. (2020) suggest that effective workplace cultures are good places to work. Such cultures feature collective leadership and everyone is living the shared values. There are safe, critical, creative learning environments and change is for the greater good and should make a difference to service users and staff. These guiding lights are a useful means of evaluating the culture of the curriculum.

ACTIVITY 6.14

Apply collective leadership principles to quality and governance structures and processes.

OBJECTIVE

To consider the final curricular outcome.

MATERIALS NEEDED

Large room, whiteboard, flipchart, art materials, markers, pens.

INSTRUCTIONS

Introduction (10 minutes)
Create a workshop and explain that the objective is to consider the final curricular outcome, using the guiding lights.

1. Invite staff to creatively express their current experience of curriculum culture (30 minutes).
2. Discuss expressions and use frameworks (guiding lights; person-centred leadership practices; contextual elements of Person-centred Practice Framework or person-centred leadership framework; person-centred relationships) to identify (30 minutes):
   ▪ which of Cardiff et al.'s (2020) guiding lights are currently evident in your setting?
   ▪ what are you doing to enable these guiding lights?
   ▪ what/who could help you further develop the guiding lights?
3. Conclude by summarising your discussion and deciding on actions.

In drawing this chapter to a close, the final activity that you are invited to complete is a personal concept analysis of 'good curriculum leadership'.

ACTIVITY 6.15

OBJECTIVE

To enable you to explore your leadership development by generating a vison of effective leadership.

MATERIALS NEEDED

Figure 6.1 concept analysis framework, computer, notepad, journal or reflective diary.

(continued)

(continued)

INSTRUCTIONS

1. Use the knowledge you have acquired through reading about (curriculum) leadership, observing leaders, creating expressions of curriculum leadership, conversing with others and reflecting on their and your own leadership, to develop your personal framework of 'good curriculum leadership', using the concept analysis framework offered in Figure 6.1.

   If you are struggling to get started, try these questions.
   - What do you hope to be as a leader? What do you fear?
   - How have you taken the lead in the past? For instance, in the school playground? What was characteristic of you taking the lead?
   - In times of uncertainty, what are your primary thoughts and reactions? Do they persist or are you able to manage them?
   - What impact would you like to achieve as a leader? What would you like to initiate/create/accomplish?
   - For what do you want to take responsibility and be held accountable?
   - What in your working environment and organisation enables you to/hinders you from taking on a leader role?

2. To keep it current and robust, we recommend you review it regularly (half yearly) to reflect and critique by yourself and then with others (be they colleague leaders or those you lead) and so enable your continued growth.

SUMMARY

- Throughout this chapter we have explored the meaning of leadership 'style' to encourage the leading of an aspect of developing a person-centred curriculum. Definitions of leadership and activities have been offered to enable a better understanding of what leadership means, what person-centred leadership looks like and how we may know that we have achieved a healthful outcome through our leadership.
- Leading curriculum development is not easy and requires navigating the challenges and tensions that exist in a workplace.
- To enable development of leadership style, knowing self as an emotionally intelligent and resonant leader and being conscious about leadership identity are imperative.
- Through undertaking and revisiting the activities offered in this chapter, it is anticipated that leadership style will be clarified and that curriculum leaders can continuously grow as persons and as leaders.

REFERENCES

Bolton, G. (2014). *Reflective Practice. Writing and Professional Development*, 4e. London: Sage.

Bolton, G. and Delderfield, R. (2018). *Reflective Practice: Writing and Professional Development*. London: Sage.

Brown, D. and McCormack, B. (2016). Exploring psychological safety as a component of facilitation within the Promoting Action Research in Health Services framework. *Journal of Clinical Nursing* 25: 2912–2932.

Brown, D. and Tropea, S. (2021). Knowing self. In: *Fundamentals of Person-centred Healthcare Practice* (ed. B. McCormack, T. McCance, C. Bulley, et al.), 34–40. Oxford: Wiley.

Cardiff, S., McCormack, B., and McCance, T. (2018). Person-centred leadership: a relational approach to leadership derived through action research. *Journal of Clinical Nursing* 27 (15-16): 3056–3069.

Cardiff, S., Sanders, K., Webester, J., and Manley, K. (2020). Guiding lights for effective workplace cultures that are also good places to work. *International Journal Practice Development* 10 (2).

Coninck, L., van Lieshout, F., van Luin, G. et al. (2023). Hoofdstuk 6: Leiderschapsidentiteit: je positie passen. In: *Stevig (leren)staan. Aan de Slag met professionele identiteit in beroep en opleiding* (ed. M. Ruijters and N. Benthum), 157–194. Paris: Management Impact.

Cook, N.F., Brown, D., O'Donnell, D. et al. (2022). The Person-centred Curriculum Framework: a universal curriculum framework for person-centred healthcare practitioner education. *International Practice Development Journal* 12 (4): 1–11.

Cummings, G.C., Grau, A.L., and Wong, C.A. (2014). Resonant leadership and workplace empowerment: the value of positive organisational cultures in reducing workplace incivility. *Nursing Economics* 32 (1): 5–16.

Cummings, G., Hewko, S., Wang, M. et al. (2018). Impact of managers' coaching conversations on staff knowledge use and performance in long-term care settings. *Worldviews on Evidence-Based Nursing* 15 (1): 62–71.

Drennan, D. (1992). *Transforming Company Culture*. London: McGraw-Hill.

Edmondson, A.C. (2012). *Teaming: How Organisations Learn, Innovate and Compete in a Knowledge Economy*. San Francisco: John Wiley & Sons.

Goleman, D. (1995). *Emotional Intelligence. Why It Can Matter More than IQ*. London: Bloomsbury Publishing.

Goleman, D., Boyatzis, R., and McKee, A. (2013). *Primal Leadership: Unleashing the Power of Emotional Intelligence*. Harvard, MA: Harvard Business Review Press.

Hardiman, M. and Dewing, J. (2014). Critical ally and critical friend: stepping stones to facilitating practice development. *International Journal of Practice Development* 4 (1).

Janssen, B. and Jacobs, G. (2018). Eigen regie en Waardigheid in de zorg: een kwestie van persoonsgerichte praktijkvoering. *Journal of Social Intervention: Theory and Practice* 27 (6): 48–64.

Jordan, J., Wade, M., and Teracino, E. (2020). Every Leader Needs to Navigate These 7 Tensions. Harvard Business Review. https://hbr.org/2020/02/every-leader-needs-to-navigate-these-7-tensions

Kouzes, J.M. and Posner, B.Z. (2017). *A Coach's Guide to Developing Exemplary Leaders: Making the Most of the Leadership Challenge and the Leadership Practices Inventory (LPI)*, 2e. New Jersey: John Wiley & Sons.

van Lieshout, F. (2013). Taking Action for Action. A study of the interplay between contextual and facilitator characteristics in developing an effective workplace culture in a Dutch hospital setting, through action research. PhD, thesis, University of Ulster, Belfast, UK.

Lynch, B., McCance, T., McCormack, B., and Brown, D. (2017). The development of the person-centred situational leadership framework: revealing the being of person-centredness in nursing homes. *Journal of Clinical Nursing* 27 (1–2): 427–440.

Lynch, B., Barron, D., and McKinlay, L. (2021). Connecting with others. In: *Fundamentals of Person-centred Healthcare Practice* (ed. B. McCormack, T. McCance, C. Bulley, et al.), 94–101. Oxford: Wiley.

Mackay, M. and Jans, C. (2022). Facilitating person-centred learning between nursing students and clinical supervisors in practice: guideline and programme development. *International Practice Development Journal* 12 (1): article 3.

Mackay, M., Jans, C., Dewing, J. et al. (2021). Enabling nursing students to have a voice in designing a learning resource to support their participation in a clinical placement. *International Practice Development Journal* 11 (2): Article 4.

Manley, K., Sanders, K., Cardiff, S., and Webster, J. (2011). Effective workplace culture: the attributes, enabling factors and consequences of a new concept. *International Journal of Practice Development* 1 (2).

Masterson, A. (2007). Community matrons: the value of knowing self (part two). *Nursing Older People* 19 (5): 29–31.

McCormack, B. and McCance, T. (ed.) (2017). *Person-centred Practice in Nursing and Health Care: Theory and Practice*. Chichester: Wiley Blackwell.

Moore, G. (2017). *Virtue at Work: Ethics for Individuals, Managers, and Organizations*. New York: Oxford University Press.

Sanders, C. (2021). 'Muchness' as the subjective experience of well-being: A participatory inquiry with nurses. PhD thesis, Queen Margaret University, Edinburgh.

Schein, E. (2010). *Organizational Culture and Leadership*, 4e. San Francisco: Jossey-Bass.

Seedhouse, D. (2017). *Thoughtful Healthcare: Ethical Awareness and Reflective Practice*. London: Sage.

Stevens, A. (2002) Archetype Revisited: An Updated Natural History of the Self. London, Brunner-Routledge.

Titchen, A., Dewing, J., and Manley, K. (2013). Getting going with facilitation skills in practice development. In: *Practice Development in Nursing and Healthcare* (ed. B. McCormack, K. Manley, and A. Titchen), 109–129. Oxford: Wiley-Blackwell.

Van Lieshout, F. (2017). Navigating organisational change: being a person-centred facilitator. In: *Person-Centred Practice in Nursing and Health Care. Theory and Practice* (ed. B. McCormack and T. McCance), 172–179. Oxford: Wiley-Blackwell.

Walker, L.O. and Avant, K.C. (2011). *Strategies for Theory Construction in Nursing*, 5e. Boston, MA: Prentice Hall.

Wang, N., Young, T., Wilhite, S., and Marczyk, G. (2011). Assessing students' emotional competence in higher education: development and validation of the widener emotional learning scale. *Journal of Psychoeducational Assessment* 29: 47–62.

Zahavi, D. (2014) Self and Other: Exploring Subjectivity, Empathy, and Shame. Oxford: Oxford University Press.

CHAPTER 7

Staff

In this chapter, we will consider the people involved in person-centred curricula and how they shape and influence the curriculum to create the conditions for learners and staff to flourish. We view staff as educators and those who support the delivery of the curriculum, and this chapter will focus on how staff teams can be developed to create, deliver and progress a person-centred curriculum. We will provide tools and resources to help address the following development themes.

- Integrating staff well-being practices in a person-centred health-care system.
- Developing a systematic approach to ongoing learning and development.
- Identifying gaps in required capabilities or resources and strategies for addressing these.

INTRODUCTION

This chapter focuses on the staff component of the Person-centred Curriculum Framework. In this framework, we define staff as:

> The general capabilities of the team with responsibility for delivering the curriculum, the skill-mix of the team and the support for staff development to deliver the curriculum, i.e. the team's make-up, its fit with the curriculum intentions and staff support to deliver curriculum outcomes.

Providing a person-centred curriculum is a complex continuing process involving knowing, doing and being (Barnett and Coate 2005). This means it is not just a case of doing, i.e. delivering the curriculum, but also a way of being underpinned by a philosophy of educational practice. This includes a clear commitment to the purpose,

Developing Person-Centred Cultures in Healthcare Education and Practice: An Essential Guide, First Edition.
Edited by Brendan McCormack.
© 2024 John Wiley & Sons Ltd. Published 2024 by John Wiley & Sons Ltd.

supported at micro-, meso- and macro-levels across education, practice and social policy areas (Dickson et al. 2020; O'Donnell et al. 2021). Those involved in designing, delivering and sustaining a person-centred curriculum should embody the values of person-centredness through an explicit commitment to the facilitation and development of learning. The staff team can include academics, practice educators, technicians and support staff, and team capabilities can be built around individuals with the necessary knowledge, skills and expertise to facilitate critical, reflexive, collaborative and engaged learning (O'Donnell et al. 2021).

In our definition of staff, we highlight how the general capabilities of the team delivering the person-centred curriculum are linked to the other components of the framework, such as skills and values. Together, these can create the conditions for staff and learners to flourish in a culture underpinned by the shared values of person-centredness. Arising from this, collaborators in developing the Person-centred Curriculum Framework identified a range of thematic actions when considering the staff that underpin a person-centred curriculum. Below are the thematic actions that will shape the content of this chapter.

1. Build the complement of capabilities of the team to embody a culture of person-centredness to enable the delivery of a person-centred curriculum.
2. Create sustainable opportunities for the academic team/education partners to develop their knowledge, skill, expertise and facilitation in critical, reflexive, collaborative learning and mentorship.
3. Ensure that job role specifications reflect the capabilities of the team needed to provide a person-centred curriculum.

FREQUENTLY ASKED QUESTIONS ABOUT STAFF

These questions (Table 7.1) are designed to help you consider what you already have as a team and what the gaps are in delivering a person-centred curriculum. The team analysis begins with understanding and agreeing on your shared values; Chapter 5 provides a process for your team to engage in this and will take you on your first steps towards understanding your team. From there, you can work to explore the curriculum you want to have, the people you need to deliver it and where the gaps may be.

TABLE 7.1   Consider the Frequently Asked Questions About Staff Teams.

Write down your initial thoughts about the capabilities of the staff responsible for delivering a person-centred curriculum. Share and discuss this with members of your team. Highlight strengths and areas that need attention and development.
- What are the general capabilities of the team responsible for delivering the person-centred curriculum? (Activity 7.1)
- What is meant by the team capability with the individual mix of staff? (Activity 7.2)
- What support, motivation and development opportunities do they need to deliver the work?

ACTIVITY 7.1

Person-centredness Simulation and Reflection

The Person-Centredness Simulation and Reflection activity is designed to immerse staff members involved in curriculum development and delivery into person-centredness principles. Through simulated scenarios, participants will gain a deeper understanding of person-centred values and practise them in real-life situations. Reflective sessions will follow the activity to uncover insights and discuss ways to implement person-centredness in their roles.

OBJECTIVES

- To provide staff with practical experience in person-centred practices.
- To facilitate the development of empathy and communication skills.
- To encourage reflection on personal and professional alignment with person-centred values.
- To identify areas for improvement and action steps for promoting a person-centred culture.

MATERIALS NEEDED

Scenario scripts and role descriptions, simulated environment (classroom or designated space), facilitator guide, reflection journals or worksheets and evaluation forms for feedback.

ACTIVITY OUTLINE

Introduction (30 minutes)

- Overview of the importance of person-centredness in education.
- Explanation of the simulation activity and its objectives.

Simulation Phase (1 hour)

Participants will engage in a series of simulated scenarios that highlight person-centred values. These scenarios may include:

- a student facing academic challenges seeking support
- a practitioner is dealing with a difficult situation involving a student
- a group project where participants must collaboratively make person-centred decisions
- participants will assume different roles in these scenarios and interact with each other as they would in real-life situations.

(continued)

(continued)

Reflection Phase (1 hour)

After each scenario, participants will gather for facilitated reflection sessions. These sessions will include:

- group discussions on what went well and what could have been done differently
- individual journalling or worksheet activities to reflect on personal experiences and feelings during the simulation
- identification of any discrepancies between actual and espoused person-centred practices.

Action Planning (30 minutes)

Participants will collectively brainstorm action steps to implement person-centred practices in their roles. This may include curriculum adjustments, communication improvements or collaborative initiatives.

Conclusion (30 minutes)

- Sharing of action plans and commitments.
- Closing remarks on the significance of embodying person-centredness.
- Distribution of resources and references for further development.

EXAMPLE OUTCOME

After participating in the Person-Centredness Simulation and Reflection activity, staff members gain practical experience applying person-centred values in various educational scenarios. They develop enhanced empathy and communication skills, allowing them to engage effectively with students and practitioners.

During the reflection phase, participants uncover insights about their alignment with person-centred principles and identify areas for improvement. They commit to action steps to promote a person-centred culture within the institution, such as revising curriculum designs to be more learner focused or initiating dialogue with colleagues about person-centred practices.

This activity catalyses cultural transformation within the institution, as staff members become advocates for person-centredness and work together to ensure that everyone is treated with dignity and respect and that their unique talents and contributions are recognised and appreciated.

ACTIVITY 7.2

Person-centred Skill Masters Workshop

The Person-Centred Skill Masters Workshop is a one-day immersive and creative experience that uniquely enhances staff teams' skills for delivering a person-centred curriculum. This workshop is designed as a role-playing adventure, where participants step into the shoes of different personas and engage in a series of scenarios to develop their skills without the need for prizes.

OBJECTIVES

- To engage staff teams in an interactive and imaginative skill development workshop.
- To encourage teamwork, empathy and skill acquisition through role-playing.
- To create a collaborative action plan for ongoing skill enhancement.
- To inspire a commitment to person-centred practices within the institution.

MATERIALS NEEDED

Facilitator(s) or workshop leader(s), role-play scenario scripts and character profiles, costume props or accessories for personas (optional), presentation materials, whiteboard and markers, evaluation forms for feedback, workshop outline

Morning (2 hours): The Person-Centred Odyssey.

- Participants are introduced to the workshop's unique role-playing format.
- Each participant selects a character profile, such as 'the struggling student', 'the educator' or 'the curriculum developer'. These character profiles represent different stakeholders in the education system, allowing participants to understand and appreciate various perspectives and challenges in implementing person-centred teaching methods.
- Participants immerse themselves in their roles and embark on a journey of person-centred scenarios.

Lunch (1 hour): Themed Picnic.

- A themed picnic lunch break where participants can relax, reflect and share their experiences from the morning session.

Afternoon (2 hours): Scenario-Based Skill Development.

- Participants engage in role-playing scenarios that require them to apply person-centred practices.
- Scenarios may include simulated student interactions, challenging teaching situations and collaborative decision-making exercises.
- Facilitators provide feedback and guidance throughout the scenarios.

(continued)

(continued)

Closing Ceremony (1 hour): Reflection and Commitment.

- Participants return to their true identities and engage in a reflective discussion.
- Each participant shares insights gained from their role-playing experiences.
- Collaboratively, the group develops an action plan for implementing person-centred practices in their roles moving forward.

Conclusion (30 minutes)

Participants leave the Person-Centred Skill Masters Workshop with a renewed commitment to person-centred education. Encourage participants to continue practising and refining their person-centred skills within the institution.

Example Outcome

After experiencing the Person-Centred Skill Masters Workshop, staff teams at your educational institution have been transformed into skilful practitioners of person-centred education. They have participated in an imaginative and engaging role-playing adventure that challenged them to apply person-centred principles in various scenarios.

The workshop fosters teamwork, empathy and a renewed dedication to person-centred practices. Staff members leave the event with a shared action plan, inspired to make person-centred education a fundamental aspect of their roles.

This creative and immersive one-day workshop enhances the institution's commitment to person-centred education, ensuring that every individual's dignity is upheld and their unique contributions are recognised and appreciated dynamically and interactively.

UNPACKING THE STRATEGIC THEMES

Essentially, the three themes can be summarised into the following areas of activity.

1. Exploring the general capabilities of the team needed to deliver a person-centred curriculum (in various contexts)
2. Creating the conditions for all team members to engage in self-development and maximise the potential for transformation.
3. Mapping and matching talent with team roles and capabilities to enable personal and team flourishing.

All persons involved with the curriculum embody the values of person-centredness through an explicit commitment to the facilitation of learning. A person-centred culture is based on a shared set of beliefs, values and behaviours in which it is evident that individuals direct and are at the centre of their own life and education (see Chapter 5).

At the core of a person-centred culture is the belief that everyone deserves to be treated with dignity and respect and to be able to live a life full of opportunities where their unique talents and contributions are recognised and appreciated. Such a culture enables effective engagement based on forming and fostering healthful relationships between all persons, with explicit values of mutual respect and understanding and respect for the person's self-determination. There also needs to be a whole system of understanding and support for person-centredness.

Therefore, staff should acknowledge and work with the whole person, be reflective and be a good communicator. To embody person-centredness, staff should have a shared understanding and the ability to reveal discrepancies between actual and espoused practices. Staff also have responsibility for being promotors of person-centredness and finding courage in challenging and changing self, their practice and their community, thus championing the conditions for everyone to flourish (Dickson et al. 2020; McCormack et al. 2021). Staff team capabilities should be built on individual professional expertise that embraces the knowledge and skill to facilitate critical, reflexive, collaborative learning.

A team leader can carry out a needs assessment to determine the capabilities of the team members/students (and practitioners) to design, deliver and evaluate a person-centred curriculum. For this reason, team leaders should identify what exists already and what learning desires are (wants). A gap analysis activity can help the team leader identify the skills the team members/students (and practitioners) need and develop a plan to recruit/acquire them. The following activity will help you explore the general capabilities of your team and consider what is needed to deliver a person-centred curriculum.

ACTIVITY 7.3

Identification of Staff Capabilities

Considering your team as a whole, identify the capabilities in your team that enable a person-centred curriculum. Write one capability in each tentacle. Having identified your team capabilities, refer to the bullet list below and identify any gaps.

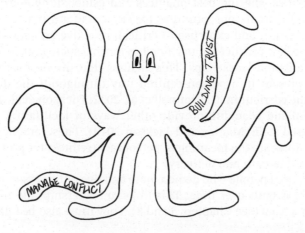

(continued)

(continued)

Specific capabilities of a person-centred team include:

- promoting person-centred ways of being
- living out person-centred ideals and values in their interactions with people
- navigating conflicting values, structures and policies
- being self-aware in interpersonal and intrapersonal relationships
- awareness of the circumstance and comprehension of how words and actions affect others or oneself
- listening attentively
- being effective communicators
- building trust
- managing conflict
- taking meaningful action in a person-centred way.

Combined with other essential skills, such as facilitation, collaboration, giving and receiving feedback, this approach can be an effective method of enabling the team to flourish (refer to Chapters 5 and 8 for further skills).

A willingness to lead self and others towards a common goal, considering the diversity of team members and individual learning and development needs, helps staff articulate and illustrate the importance of person-centredness in professional practice, curriculum development and delivery.

Investment in staff development, with particular attention to team members' diversity and individual learning and development needs, enables the necessary attributes to deliver the person-centred curriculum. Leaders should recognise and create opportunities for the staff team to develop their knowledge, skills and expertise in critical, reflexive, collaborative learning through staff induction, peer-supported activities, sharing best practices and establishing communities of practice. Staff can also create opportunities for students (and practitioners) to develop their knowledge, skill and expertise in critical, reflexive and collaborative learning through sharing best practices in partnership forums such as curriculum design and curriculum evaluation workshops. This ensures that the necessary person-centred attributes are present in a person-centred way throughout the design and implementation of the curriculum (O'Donnell et al. 2022; Dickson et al. 2020). Peer learning, mentorship and coaching provide other ways of facilitating the development of person-centred staff (Manley and Jackson 2019). These practices enable staff to articulate and illustrate the meaning of person-centredness for professional practice, curriculum development and delivery.

Staff teams need people who demonstrate and live out a person-centred approach, so team culture is built over time. This links *to* leadership and new people's skills when they join a team (see Chapters 5 and 8). They must also be followers, and teams must consider their leadership continuity and influence over time. When forming a team, the team leader should involve the members in a skill-oriented manner (a perfect mix of skills in the team/community) and pay attention to the diversity of skills within the team.

In order to provide a person-centred curriculum, it is important to have clearly defined roles and responsibilities within the team (e.g. educators, professional support staff, managers and leaders). When each team member has a clearly defined role, there is no confusion, communication problems or continuity interruptions in person-centred facilitation. It also helps to create person profiles (talents and needs) shared in multiple, pragmatic/realistic ways throughout all levels of the organisation (e.g. team/community members sharing amongst themselves). Clearly defined roles in the team enable leaders to know their team/community skills and recognise an opportunity for a team/community member to grow their knowledge, skills and expertise.

Examples of the mix of skills that staff involved in person-centred curricula should have are:

- being responsive to feedback through individual and team practices
- developing psychologically safe learning environments to create the conditions to be both challenging and supportive, and valuing individual personhood
- creating person-centred environments for everyone to flourish
- fostering relationships that are reciprocal, respectful, inclusive and collaborative with other teams and stakeholders
- supporting or coaching learners in choosing their pathway in a flexible curriculum.

We will now consider how staff talents and capabilities can match roles.

A curriculum does not just 'happen'. People enable the design, delivery and continued improvement of a curriculum. Suppose we want to educate future person-centred healthcare practitioners through a person-centred curriculum. In that case, we are compelled to look at the current 'staff situation' and possibly reconfigure individual and/or job tasks and responsibilities so that existent talents and expertise are adequately utilised, gaps identified and developmental and/or recruitment activities instigated. We may achieve this by moving away from thinking solely about 'job descriptions', which usually contain multiple roles, responsibilities and tasks, and focus on individual roles and responsibilities, with or without associated tasks.

Activity 7.4 below, with the associated tools (Tables 7.2–7.6), could offer a starting point in ensuring that the staff make-up fits curriculum needs to meet ambitions. Imagine what could happen if we created a unique (and dynamic) job description per individual with a mix of roles/responsibilities and tasks matching their talents and learning needs. This is a different approach from searching for an individual to fit a pre-set job description. What each person then leads and performs could contribute more to the whole curriculum than when they conform to the job description in their human resources file.

ACTIVITY 7.4

Staff Requirements

PHASE 1: WHAT DO WE NEED?

Your curriculum may have a beautifully worded vision, mission and/or aims. But does it have an inventory of the roles/responsibilities and tasks needed to fulfil these ambitions? If not, then that may be an innovative starting point. Regardless of who takes on which role/responsibility or performs which task, the question is whether we know what needs to be done. The following two steps can be worked through to develop an overview of what is needed (see Table 7.2). Steps 1 and 2 can be repeated for curriculum design, delivery and (continuous) development separately or collectively, depending on the size/scope of the team and curriculum.

STEP 1: MAKE AN INVENTORY OF ROLES/RESPONSIBILITIES AND TASKS

1. Call up all the job descriptions involved in the delivery of a curriculum. Pull out all the individual tasks and roles/responsibilities. Place them in two piles: one for 'tasks' ('do' activities) and another for 'roles/responsibilities' (leading/accounting for an area or facet of the curriculum).
2. Call together a group of staff currently holding various positions within the curriculum team. There should be a mix of (educational and practice setting) management, educational and administration staff, and learners.
3. Invite participants to review the pile of 'roles/responsibilities' for completeness. Add missing roles/responsibilities and then try to reduce them to a minimum. Some roles/responsibilities may be so similar that they warrant clustering into one role/responsibility. The final overview (see column 1 of Table 7.2) should be undisputed, i.e. consensus (agreement by all) or consent (no insurmountable objections) has been achieved.
4. Working with the same or new group of staff, review the pile of 'tasks' for completeness, cluster where possible and seek consensus or consent for the final overview (see column 2 of Table 7.2).
5. Finally, the inventory (Table 7.2) of roles/responsibilities and tasks should be member-checked with a wider audience.

TABLE 7.2 Inventory of Roles, Responsibilities and Tasks Required to Design, Deliver and Develop the Curriculum.

Role and responsibility descriptor	Tasks
1.	1.
2.	2.
3.	3.

STEP 2: IDENTIFYING CAPABILITIES (EXPERTISE AND TALENTS) NEEDED TO FULFIL RESPONSIBILITIES AND TASKS

1. Call together a heterogeneous group of staff active in the curriculum. Invite them to discuss and determine which expertise (knowledge) and/or talents (skills) a person needs to fulfil each role/responsibility. Again, consensus or consent should be sought.
2. Working with the same or new group of staff, identify the expertise (knowledge) and/or talents (skills) a person needs to fulfil each task. Cluster where possible and seek consensus or consent for the final overview.
3. The inventory (see Table 7.3) of talents and expertise for each role/responsibility and task can be member-checked with a wider audience.

PHASE 2: WHO CAN LEAD WHAT?

The assumption here is that a mix of knowledge and skills is needed to fulfil those roles/responsibilities and tasks for the curriculum's design, delivery and continued improvement. Another assumption is that no two individuals are identical in their talents (what they competently and seemingly effortlessly execute) and expertise (specific knowledge and/or skills). So, the chance is small that the talents and expertise of any one person will match and fulfil all those needed for the range of tasks associated with certain roles/responsibilities named in any job description. The following two steps can be worked through to develop an overview of the team's

TABLE 7.3 Overview of Roles, Responsibilities and Tasks Needed, With Corresponding Talents and Expertise.

Role and responsibility descriptor	Talents and expertise needed to fulfil role/responsibility	Tasks	Talents and expertise needed to fulfil a task
1	a.	1	a.
	b.		b.
	c.		c.
	d.		d.
	e.		e.
2	a.	2	a.
	b.		b.
	c.		c.
	d.		d.
	e.		e.
3	a.	3	a.
	b.		b.
	c.		c.
	d.		d.
	e.		e.

(continued)

(continued)

TABLE 7.4   The Staff Expertise, Talent and Learning Needs Inventory.

Staff member	Self-identified talents and expertise	Extra (observed/ fed back) talents and expertise	Self-identified learning needs
A.	1. 2. 3.	1. 2. 3.	1. 2. 3.
B.	1. 2. 3.	1. 2. 3.	1. 2. 3.
C.	1. 2. 3.	1. 2. 3.	1. 2. 3.
D.	1. 2. 3.	1. 2. 3.	1. 2. 3.
E.	1. 2. 3.	1. 2. 3.	1. 2. 3.

current capabilities and learning needs (see Table 7.4) and match these to the roles, responsibilities and tasks identified in the previous phase (see Tables 7.5 and 7.6) needs. Steps 1 and 2 can be repeated for curriculum design, delivery and (continuous) development separately or collectively, depending on the size/scope of the team and curriculum.

STEP 1: IDENTIFYING STAFF CAPABILITIES (EXPERTISE AND TALENTS) AND LEARNING NEEDS

1. Invite every team member to personally/individually identify their top five talents and specific knowledge and skills (expertise). If they find this challenging, ask them to describe as accurately as possible a situation in which the time seemed to fly, and it cost them little energy to get started or keep going and in which they had a good feeling of 'job well done' by the end, even though they may have felt tired. They can identify what they did/used to fulfil the job. These then become their talents, including specific knowledge and skills. They may also refer to feedback others gave them: 'I am often told that ....; People tend to compliment me on my ...'. They may not even have been aware that others saw these actions as exceptional. Talent identification can also be helped by offering examples, such as:
   - communicating effectively with skills such as oral/written/non-verbal communication, active listening, presentation, public speaking, negotiation, persuasion and discussion skills, etc.

TABLE 7.5 Matching Roles and Responsibilities to Staff Members with Required Talents and Expertise.

Role and responsibility descriptor	Talents and expertise needed to fulfil role/ responsibility	Staff whose talents and expertise match the role/ responsibility need	Definite matches
1.	i.	a. ___/___/___	1.
	ii.	b. ___/___/___	2.
	iii.	c. ___/___/___	
	iv.	d. ___/___/___	
	v.	e. ___/___/___	
2.	i.	a. ___/___/___	1.
	ii.	b. ___/___/___	2.
	iii.	c. ___/___/___	
	iv.	d. ___/___/___	
	v.	c. ___/___/___	
3.	i.	a. ___/___/___	1.
	ii.	b. ___/___/___	2.
	iii.	c. ___/___/___	
	iv.	d. ___/___/___	
	v.	e. ___/___/___	

TABLE 7.6 Matching Tasks with Staff Members' Required Talents and Expertise.

Task descriptor	Talents and expertise needed to fulfil a task	Staff whose talents and expertise match the task requirements	Definite matches
1.	i.	a. ___/___/___	1.
	ii.	b. ___/___/___	2.
	iii.	c. ___/___/___	
	iv.	d. ___/___/___	
	v.	e. ___/___/___	
2.	i.	a. ___/___/___	1.
	ii.	b. ___/___/___	2.
	iii.	c. ___/___/___	
	iv.	d. ___/___/___	
	v.	e. ___/___/___	
3.	i.	a. ___/___/___	1.
	ii.	b. ___/___/___	2.
	iii.	c. ___/___/___	
	iv.	d. ___/___/___	
	v.	e. ___/___/___	

(continued)

(continued)

- working digitally with skills such as navigating MS Office programs, social media, database management, troubleshooting, equipment installation and configuration, fast typing, etc.
- managing processes/leading people with skills such as goal planning, time management, risk management, decisiveness, action planning, conflict resolution, team building, etc.
- leading people through skills such as relationship building, enthusing, creativity, strategic thinking, facilitating, etc.
- problem solving with analytical and critical thinking skills, data gathering and analysis, attention to detail, theory and research exploration, etc.
- organising through skills such as spatial awareness, scheduling, delegation, monitoring, networking, etc.
- hospitality with skills such as creating attractive/welcoming environments and first impressions; positivity; organisational knowledge (who's who); sympathising; chasing.

2. Invite staff to seek feedback from (at least) two other team members about their top five talents and expert knowledge and skills list. It may well be that some talents or expertise remain within their blind spot. Seeking feedback will help raise self-awareness of these and those talents and expertise team members see as vital for effective and efficient curriculum design, delivery and development. If the talent list expands beyond five, this is not a problem, but it may be good to rank them.

3. Now, invite staff to identify their learning needs; for example, which talents, knowledge or skills would they like to develop? These may be talents or areas of expertise that currently do not score so high in the ranking or areas they are interested in and would like to develop for personal/professional growth.

STEP 2: IDENTIFYING WHO CAN BEST DO WHAT IN LIGHT OF THEIR PERSONAL EXPERTISE, TALENTS AND LEARNING NEEDS

One could consider various methods when matching persons (and their capabilities or learning needs) to roles, responsibilities and tasks. A few are offered below but can easily be expanded or adapted to meet local preferences and possibilities. The essence of this step is to enable self-determination of how each person wants to use their talents, expertise and learning needs when contributing to the curriculum's design, delivery and development.

STEP 3: MATCHING PERSONS (AND THEIR CAPABILITIES OR LEARNING NEEDS) TO ROLES, RESPONSIBILITIES AND TASKS

Run a workshop: a workshop where staff work in (homogeneous) duos or quads to discuss each other's talents, expertise and learning needs before individually volunteering to adopt specific roles, responsibilities and tasks identified in Table 7.3.

1. *Poster and volunteering*: on a poster, identify the roles/responsibilities/tasks, talents and expertise matrix. Invite people to volunteer for as many 'vacancies' as they feel capable of fulfilling. It is also useful if they indicate whether they possess the required talent or expertise already or if it is a learning need. This 'poster and volunteering' method could also be done digitally by creating an Excel file and making the file accessible for completion through a local/organisational platform.
2. *Recommend colleagues*: as well as staff volunteering, the team can be invited to recommend colleagues based on their observations of or belief in a colleague's talents, expertise or learning need.

PHASE 3: WHO DO WE NEED TO RECRUIT?

Having identified roles, responsibilities and tasks and matched existing staff capabilities to them, there may still be some roles, responsibilities or tasks with no one to fulfil them. Possible explanations could be that requirements exceed capacity (staff do not have the 'space' to fulfil so many roles, responsibilities or tasks) or exceed capabilities (no one has the expertise or talent(s) needed). When requirements exceed capabilities, a team can look at learning needs first (step 1). When capacity is an issue, new members must be recruited from outside the team (step 2). Steps 1 and 2 may be worked through each time a staff member leaves the team.

STEP 1: RESOLVING VACANCIES

- Create a small working group to identify gaps within Tables 7.5 and 7.6.
- For each 'vacancy', check column 4 of Table 7.4 for potential candidates.
- Consult potential candidates to determine their interest in taking on the role, responsibility or task their learning needs would match and explore what is needed to enable them to grow into the position.
- Set in process learning development plans using support from team leaders, HR consultants and other relevant resources within the organisation (or beyond).
- Update Tables 7.5 and 7.6.

STEP 2: RECRUITING NEW TALENTS AND EXPERTISE

- Create a small working group to identify gaps in Tables 7.5 and 7.6.
- Collate the mix of roles, responsibilities, tasks and the required expertise and talents.
- Design a colourful and creative vacancy text/advertisement attracting someone with many of the required capabilities and desires to fulfil the named roles, responsibilities and tasks.
- Be explicit in making potential candidates aware of the supportive environment and space to 'learn' some capabilities they may not have.

Leaders should be attentive to optimum staff–student ratios and diversity of skills to realise effective teaching, with facilitation at the heart of teaching, learning and assessment practices (O'Donnell et al. 2022). The OECD (2022) suggests the average student-to-academic staff ratio is 15:1 in higher education. Consider if this is the case in your organisation by completing the following activity.

ACTIVITY 7.5

Determine Your Student: Staff Ratio

The ratio of students to academic staff is obtained by dividing the number of full-time equivalent (FTE) students at a given level of education by the number of full-time equivalent academic staff at that level. Work out your actual staff:student ratio and consider the implications of this for the staff team and learners in terms of supporting a person-centred curriculum.

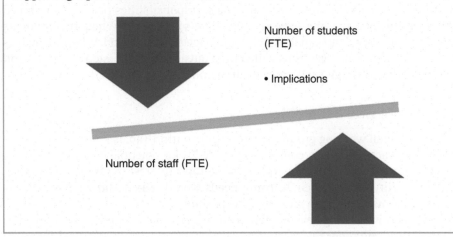

Number of students (FTE)

• Implications

Number of staff (FTE)

INTRAORGANISATIONAL LEARNING AND DEVELOPMENT FOR STAFF

Induction Programmes

Induction programmes are designed to support new members of staff joining the team and can vary in content and duration, depending on the organisation and the individual. While there may be a focus on the practicalities of settling into an organisation, a focused induction programme can reflect the culture of the organisation and what it values. This can shape the individual's experience of a person-centred culture, and every interaction will influence this. The opportunity to consider the educational philosophy underpinning the person-centred curriculum, the language and behaviours used, and how the curriculum is delivered will provide a foundation for new team members to adapt and develop their practice and embody person-centredness. A good induction programme will identify a support buddy or mentor for each new team member who can help identify their learning needs, develop a learning plan and implement it.

The length of time for induction programmes can vary depending on the context, but it can be useful to break it down into manageable timeframes to achieve particular milestones, for example, the first week, first month, first three months, six months and so on.

ACTIVITY 7.6

Induction Programme Design

Review your organisation's current induction arrangements/programme and identify how it meets the needs of new members of the staff team. Then identify what would enhance the induction programme to align it with person-centredness.

Current induction	Person-centred induction
▪	▪
▪	▪
▪	▪
▪	▪

Once you have identified what is required in an induction programme, you can create an induction plan and break it down into the immediate basics, getting started and further development. This can be matched to a timeline that can vary depending on the person and the context but is often over 3–6 months. Below is a suggested time frame and activities with expectations.

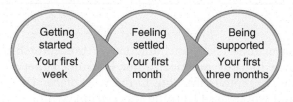

Each circle can be expanded to identify what it might look like.

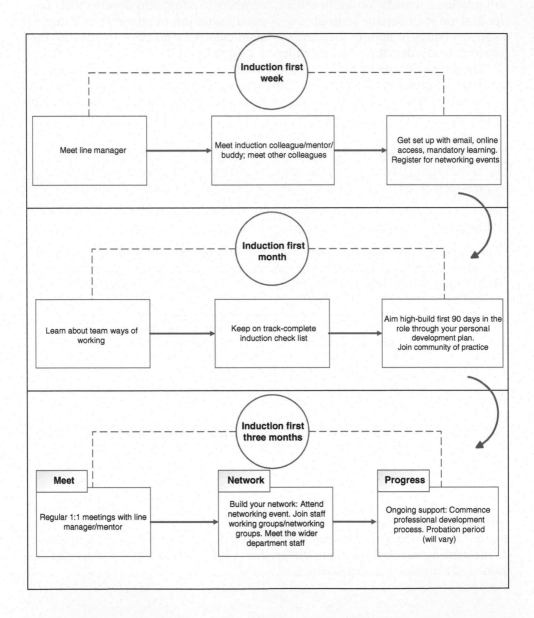

Once you have undertaken an induction or preceptorship programme and gained confidence in your practice, other learning supervision roles can be offered to enable continuous learning in the workplace. These include mentorship, coaching and work-based learning supervision. While these roles overlap in the helping styles and processes they use, they have different functions, which we show below.

Mentorship

Mentorship takes a longer-term view and helps you see the bigger picture of your career and what you want to work towards. Your mentor is like a companion on your learning journey, offering you guidance and support concerning your work. Mentors:

- help you reflect on your practice
- help you learn through role-modelling and sharing the knowledge they have acquired through learning on the job and any work-based learning they might have undertaken
- offer you justified praise and celebrate your achievements and successes, however small
- give you feedback, ask enabling questions to help you discover your 'blind spots', analyse your issues and problems and work towards solutions and making good decisions
- provide emotional and moral support
- offer advice about your career, develop social contacts and build networks
- introduce you to helpful contacts.

ACTIVITY 7.7

Getting to Know Your Mentor/Mentee

Arrange to meet for coffee to get to know each other in an informal setting. Share career backgrounds and talk about other informal topics – hobbies, family, plans for the weekend. This will help get to know the person and build trust. Arrange to meet regularly (weekly at first, then two to three weekly). Depending on personal preference, this could be in a more formal setting or in an informal way. You might want to walk or meet in an office setting. Set some clear and realistic goals and targets to review progress. Plan some activities such as job shadowing, attending relevant meetings together, creating networks and identifying organisational training and development opportunities.

While the activity above refers to individual mentors/mentees, small group mentoring can be as effective, so consider bringing several new staff together to share feedback and observe. This will allow them to connect with each other, and share experiences and ideas in a facilitated, structured way.

Coaching

Coaching focuses on helping you to improve some particular aspect of your practice. A coach helps you draw on your resources to improve your knowledge, know-how, skills and competencies rather than introducing you to new ones. A coaching style is thus recognised by collaborating, negotiating, involving and explaining processes.

The coach's role is to help others reveal to themselves the knowledge embedded in them and their practices that are invisible to them (and maybe others, too). The coach helps them to bring it to the surface and develop it further to bring about sustained learning and improvement. This is done mainly by asking enabling questions and high challenge/high support to help the person learn from their resources. The coach will check that the person can successfully transfer their new learning to other situations. There may be times when the person is out of their depth, in other words has no inner resources or knowledge to draw on, and this is where it is necessary to switch to a more directing, mentoring style where the coach suggests ideas, structures the learning, shares what they know and guides the learner.

Coaching can take many forms, and the activity below is one example of how to develop educational practice and enable human flourishing.

ACTIVITY 7.8

Person-centred, Peer-to-peer Shadowing

Shadowing here is defined as a method whereby one person (the shadower) walks in the shadow of another person (the shadowee) for a time, gathering and processing information that can then be fed back if and when desired. The shadower uses their senses to collect data about the shadowee within their natural (working) environment. As a shadower, your presence should be overt but as unobtrusive as possible, and your feeding back of observations should be aligned to the values underpinning person-centredness: respect for personhood and the right to self-determination, alongside mutual respect and understanding.

Traditionally, shadowing has been used as a learning method for learners/newcomers to understand current practices and culture by observing a more experienced colleague (Lalleman et al. 2017). However, peer-to-peer shadowing can also be used as a practice development method when an individual's practice and the workplace culture are observed, observations fed back, and critically dialogued to enable human flourishing and person-centred practice (Dewing et al. 2014). Person-centred practice is relevant to educational practice when viewed as the continuous and collaborative forming of relationships and structures within care, learning and working environments with an authentic intent of enabling mutual understanding while respecting each person and their right to self-determination (Jacobs and Jansen 2018; McCormack et al. 2021).

What is Shadowing Used for Here?

Peer-to-peer shadowing in an educational environment can have multiple goals.

- *Enabling professional development*: when the shadower and shadowee can reflect on the meaning of practice observations.
- *Fostering quality/practice improvement*: when observations are fed back, critically dialogued and result in practice improvement planning.

- *On-boarding for new staff members*: allows them to observe and critically question current practices before adopting observed behaviours and routines.
- *Strengthening weak(er) relationships among staff members*: the shadowing process requires a willingness to show vulnerability, mindfully and respectfully offering/ receiving feedback, and seeking shared understanding between the shadower and shadowee.

How Can It Be Conducted?

Shadowing is not an exercise that can be executed 'quickly' or without careful thought with regard to each phase of the process and the potential effect on all stakeholders (all who may be affected/influenced by the process or outcome). Lack of reflection before action could result in more damage than good. To structure the shadowing process, we suggest using the four-phase model of Buchanan et al. (2013): getting in (prepared), getting on, getting out, getting back.

Phase One: Getting Prepared

This preparatory phase entails negotiating who (to shadow), what (to focus on), when-where-how (to conduct it) and why (shadowing is considered a suitable method for intended goals). The motivation for engaging in peer-to-peer shadowing may be extrinsic (e.g. local policy requiring regular peer-to-peer shadowing) or intrinsic (e.g. a personal desire to shadow/be shadowed). Either way, you and the shadowee need to find each other and negotiate what, when, where, how and why.

Buchanan et al. (2013) advise allowing sufficient time to organise the 'getting on' phase; be mindful of who you approach and why; be able to articulate a 'win/win' scenario; be observant for and sympathetic towards reservations, respect the need for time to consider the offer; if unfamiliar, be explicit about purpose and the shadowing process, and include the observation feedback process.

While the 'basic shadowing agreement' (see Table 7.7) is a good starting point to negotiating the shadowing process, we advise building rapport first through general conversation and exploring each other's hopes, fears and expectations about the shadowing process. This will create time, space and a sense of psychological safety for sharing something you or the other may initially find uncomfortable or not be aware of until you start engaging in a conversation about shadowing. Starting immediately with the agreement document and only sticking to that could prevent such issues from arising or being shared – for instance, concerns about how observations are documented and saved or how observations are shared and dialogued. Issues are often personal and may vary per shadowing session. We therefore advise differentiating between 'general' and 'extra/session specific' do's/don'ts within the agreement plan (see Table 7.7), which should be reviewed before each session.

Phase Two: Getting On

Getting on is not just about 'getting on with the task at hand'. It also encompasses 'getting on with the people involved'. In line with the values underlying person-centred practice, you should return to, review and affirm the agreement each shadowing

TABLE 7.7 Basic Shadowing Agreement Plan.

The following agreement has been collaboratively completed by:

Shadowee:...................(*insert name here*)

Shadower:...................(*insert name here*)

The purpose/aim of the shadowing is:

For shadowee:................... *(insert hopes/expectations here)*

For shadower:................... *(insert hopes/expectations here)*

General do's and don'ts:

✓ ....(*list here*)

Ø ....(*list here*)

Extra general agreements:

■ ....(*insert here*)

■ ....(*insert here*)

■ ....(*insert here*)

Shadowing sessions	Date:........... From:........hrs To:...........hrs Location:...........	Date:........... From:........hrs To:...........hrs Location:...........	Date:........... From:........hrs To:...........hrs Location:...........
Preparation of setting	By:........... Specific attention to:...........	By:........... Specific attention to:...........	By:........... Specific attention to:...........
Specific do's and don'ts	✓ .... Ø	✓ .... Ø	✓ .... Ø ....
Feedback session	Date:........... From:........hrs To:...........hrs Location:...........	Date:........... From:........hrs To:...........hrs Location:...........	Date:........... From:........hrs To:...........hrs Location:...........
Extra specific agreements			

session. The worlds we inhabit are not static and circumstances may have changed for you/the shadowee/the context. While you are not shadowing others within the setting, you will be observing interactions between the shadowee and others within the setting. These people should also receive respectful explanation of the process and consent should be sought for documenting interactions so that anonymity is maximised. Ideally, the shadowee should obtain their consent.

As well as the overall purpose/aim, it is advisable to negotiate specific areas of practice (topics) to be observed, per session. The list of topics should not extend your speed or capacity to observe and then document your observations in sufficient detail. Using theoretical frameworks can also help you identify specific/relevant areas of interest. Frameworks potentially useful for educational practice include the Person-centred Practice Framework (McCormack et al. 2021), the Person-centred Leadership Framework (Cardiff et al. 2018) and the Critical Ally/Friend/Companion Frameworks (Hardiman and Dewing 2014; Titchen 2004).

You may find the observation tool in Table 7.8 useful. However, if you feel more comfortable working with a notebook or electronic device such as an i-pad, do not hesitate to use them. While you are busy documenting what you sense, clarifying questions will undoubtedly arise and should be noted for a later/convenient moment. You should be careful to only ask clarifying questions at this stage and not engage in a critical dialogue about observations until you have had opportunity to process your notes.

While the focus of shadowing entails observing the shadowee in their educational practice, you should also be mindful and reflexive on your own shadowing practice. Your presence may influence the shadowee and how they engage in their practice, whether that be giving a lecture, facilitating a workgroup or supervising/mentoring a learner in a healthcare setting.

The thought of shadowing a colleague does not often seem like hard work but the reality is often more tiring than expected. We therefore advise beginners to start with 15–20-minute sessions, particularly in busy environments. These can then be extended in length as you become accustomed to/more proficient in the process.

TABLE 7.8 Observation Tool for Peer-to-Peer Shadowing.

Shadowee:	_____	Location:	_____
Shadower:	_____		
Observation topics/foci:	_____	Date and times:	_____
	_____		
	_____		
	_____		
Time	**Observations** *(I see . . .; I hear . . .; I smell . . .; I imagine . . .)*	**Clarifying questions**	

Phase Three: Getting Out

Shadowing can be intense, and sharing fosters intimacy within working relationships. Care should therefore be taken not to end shadowing sessions or the shadowing period abruptly. A useful rule of thumb is to 'check out' by reviewing how the shadowee feels at that moment in time, the shadowing process they leave behind and the future awaiting them. It is also respectful to agree and keep to agreed time frames (start/stop times and dates) and confirm the next meeting dates and times before you actually leave the setting. Do not forget to reiterate the possibility of 'in-between' contact moments if and when they are needed.

The feeding back of observations may be conducted at the end of the agreed shadowing session, or you may need some time to review your notes before feeding back your observations. Therefore, the 'getting back' phase below includes guidelines for the feedback process.

Phase Four: Getting Back

Getting back may be to gather more information or to offer your observations for shadowee reflection, with or without a critical dialogue, depending on their preference. Either way, dates and times need to be agreed, and a suitable space offering some privacy found. Getting back means that you have had time to review your observations and then think about and structure what you want to feed back. The intention should be explicit and may need to be reaffirmed: 'We're here so that I can feed back my observations that will hopefully help you to continue and grow in the areas we agreed beforehand'. Check that the shadowee is open to receiving feedback before starting.

During or after the feedback process, the shadowee may want to make notes about what was said, insights gained and developmental actions. This can also be done in co-creation. The feedback and action planning tool below in Table 7.9 will help you prepare observations you want to feed back (column 1), collaboratively identify insights gained during the critical dialogue about the observations (column 2), and plan actions for professional growth (column 3).

The following guiding principles for giving and receiving feedback (Dewing et al. 2014) will also help the process.

1. Practise beforehand what and how you want to say what you want to feed back.
2. Ensure your facts are right and there is a mix of 'claims' and 'concerns'.
3. Be non-judgemental and neutral in your descriptions of their behaviour. Restrict yourself to observed behaviour and do not wander into their personhood.

TABLE 7.9 Feedback Action Planning Tool.

Shadowee: _____	Date and location: _____
Shadower: _____	_____
Key observations	**(Shadowee) Insights**	**Action to be taken**

4. Encourage the shadowee to share their own self-assessment first before offering your observations.
5. Engage authentically.
6. Be sympathetically present.
7. Offer non-judgemental feedback which is truthful (as determined by you), direct and constructive.
8. Be future oriented and think 'with' (not 'for') the shadowee in determining insights, whether or not and how to move forward (action planning).
9. Offer follow-up support.
10. Offer space for the shadowee to give you feedback on how you gave feedback, and how it could be more effective.

The following guiding principles for a critical dialogue may also be of help.

1. A dialogue aims to achieve mutual understanding and acceptance, which is not necessarily consensus about conclusions.
2. A dialogue is 'critical' when assumptions are questioned and 'power over' is challenged.
3. Both you and the shadowee need to feel comfortable in order to share and question authentically.
4. Pace the dialogue so that there is time for thoughtful reflection.
5. Listen 'actively' and 'hear' what is being said. Try not to let yourself be distracted by your own thoughts and intentions.
6. Show your presence through non-verbal as well as verbal communication.
7. Remain goal oriented and avoid diverging into areas outside the agreed topics/focus.
8. Ask for clarity for things you do not understand and if there is anything not being said.
9. Respect responses to questions and personal choices.
10. Ensure that there is space to explore the topics' and observations' physical, psychological, social and spiritual aspects.

Curriculum Design

Collaboratively designing a curriculum can be seen as a form of professional development (Saroyan and Trigwell 2015), where staff share knowledge, exchange perspectives and solve challenges (Noben et al. 2022). The activity below is a good starting point to engage stakeholders in curriculum design and promote professional development of those involved, including learners and staff.

Curriculum Co-design Workshops

Identify and bring key stakeholders and staff together in a world café-style forum. Assign people to groups of 5–6 to consider what's working/what's not working in the curriculum. A facilitator can keep the discussion broad enough to cover the following topics and use prompt cards. Ask each group to write their contribution on flipchart paper during discussions under the following suggested themes.

- Consider the whole student journey from pre-induction to graduation/ employment.
- Consider the learning, teaching and assessment approaches integrated into the curriculum and ensure authentic assessment.
- Consider any extracurricular activities that contribute to a person-centred curriculum.
- How does timetabling/course structure/student workload align with person-centred curriculum and culture?
- What are the employability prospects for graduates from this curriculum? Does the curriculum offer work-based placement? Are workplace colleagues involved in curriculum design and delivery?
- How are pastoral care and student support processes evident in the curriculum?
- What research learning, support and opportunities are available in the curriculum?
- Is interdisciplinary learning integrated into the curriculum?
- What are the design challenges?

Allocate enough time so each theme can be considered and key points recorded on the flipchart. Each group will give feedback on one or two themes, and the facilitator will clarify where necessary and identify with the whole group what is important for the person-centred curriculum.

Curriculum and staff development should be considered as one process (Cowen et al. 2004). Staff development and well-being will be reflected in the learner experience so investment in staff development and well-being should be systems-wide and a core function of the organisation. Reflecting on the experience of designing and delivering a person-centred curriculum are useful learning and development tools for those involved in developing and delivering the curriculum.

How is Critical Reflexive Collaborative Learning Facilitated?

Critical reflexive learning is one way of developing and maintaining person-centred staff (Manley and Jackson 2019). Critical reflexive learning can be facilitated and self-facilitated, involving formal and informal tools/activities. To develop a robust skill mix in the team, it is valuable to engage in group activities where staff can learn and reflect together in safe spaces. Group cohesion is important for establishing positive workplace relations (Masimula et al. 2023) and leaders should support different activities and motivate staff to share/play on their strengths and motivations. That way, staff on different levels can be mentors and learn from each other. You may find Activity 7.9 useful to engage groups of staff in healthful conversations in a psychologically safe space (see also Chapter 5).

ACTIVITY 7.9

Healthful Coffee/Lunch Break Conversations

- Agree to have coffee/lunch with one or more colleagues.
  - The first time you meet, you may begin with this opening question: 'What does happiness at work mean to you at the moment?'
  - As you and your colleagues feel more comfortable, you may invite them to choose the cards identified in the squares below in different coloured blocks.
- Pose the question and engage in conversation.
- Closing questions could be:
  - 'What did this conversation do for you?'
  - 'Are there any other topics you can think of/questions we could ask about healthful cultures?'

Do you feel connected to the curriculum/ organisation? How would we notice this?	Does feeling connected (to the curriculum) contribute to your happiness at work? How would we notice that?	How/In what ways do you feel connected to others in the curriculum?	What do you think about the communi- cation within the curricu- lum?
What does connection mean to you when you think about the curriculum? Is it important for you?	What do you think of the connec- tion between you and your manager?	Does your man- ager give you a feeling of trust? What does your manager trust you in?	When do you dare to ask for help? Do you dare to ask this always and from everyone?
Do you dare to show your vulnerability? How would we know?	What does trust in the workplace/ curriculum mean to you?	Do you feel free to express your own opinion? Can you give an example?	Do you dare give others feedback? How do you give it in a good way?
When do you notice that you are doing mean- ingful work?	Do you feel your work contributes to something beautiful, good or important?	What gives you satisfaction at work?	How often do you feel you have been busy and done good work?

(continued)

(continued)

Are your talents utilised? How do you notice that?	Can you develop yourself sufficiently? How do you notice that?	What does autonomy mean for you?	Are your ideas or opinions listened to? How do you notice that?
Do you enjoy your work? How do you notice that?	Is there enough laughter in the workplace? Is that important for your work happiness?	What does appreciation mean to you?	Is appreciation for your work important to you? Why?
Are you recognised for what you do? Are you recognised enough?	In what way do you like to be appreciated? Why?	From whom do you receive the most appreciation? What does that look like?	Is your effort appreciated? How do you notice that?

LEGEND

Questions about:

Connectedness/ Engagement	Trust	Meaning	Fulfilment
Competency	Autonomy	Pleasure	Appreciation

How Do We Know That We are Developing Staff Who are Person-centred Practitioners?

To evaluate the development and flourishing of staff and the team, it is important to assess the ongoing and final progress/outcomes (Activity 7.10). The progress/outcomes can be measured using a variety of sources, some of which are indicated below.

- Peer feedback (see shadowing activity above).
- Staff turnover measures.
- Learner outcomes – graduate outcomes data.
- Feedback about graduates from stakeholders.
- Learner feedback and ongoing evaluation.
- Ongoing process and progress evaluation that is made visible to team members, for example in posters on notice boards or monthly newsletters.
- Annual recruitment data.

ACTIVITY 7.10

'Flourish-O-Meter': Evaluating Staff and Team Development

The 'Flourish-O-Meter' is an engaging and interactive activity designed to assess the development and flourishing of staff and teams in your educational institution. This activity encourages staff members to collaboratively evaluate progress and outcomes using various sources, fostering a culture of continuous improvement.

OBJECTIVES

1. To evaluate the development and flourishing of staff and teams through a multi-source assessment approach.
2. To promote teamwork and collaboration in the assessment process.
3. To identify areas for improvement and action steps based on assessment findings.
4. To enhance transparency and communication within the team.

MATERIALS NEEDED

Assessment templates (e.g. feedback forms, survey questionnaires), presentation materials, whiteboard and markers, notice boards or space for posters, newsletter template (electronic or printed) and access to relevant data and feedback sources.

ACTIVITY OUTLINE

Introduction (30 minutes).

- Welcome and overview of the 'Flourish-O-Meter' activity's purpose and objectives.
- Explanation of the importance of multi-source assessment for development and flourishing.

ASSESSMENT STATIONS (2 HOURS)

Participants rotate through assessment stations, each focusing on a different source of assessment.

1. Peer feedback station: participants provide and receive peer feedback based on their observations and experiences.
2. Staff turnover station: review and discuss staff turnover data, identifying trends or concerns.
3. Learner outcomes station: analyse graduate outcomes data and identify areas of strength and improvement.
4. Stakeholder feedback station: examine feedback from stakeholders about graduates and the institution's performance.

(continued)

(continued)

5. Learner feedback station: review learner feedback and ongoing evaluation data.
6. Process and progress evaluation station: evaluate ongoing processes and progress and create visual posters or content for newsletters.
7. Recruitment data station: analyse annual recruitment data to assess the institution's ability to attract and retain talent.

COLLABORATIVE DISCUSSION (1 HOUR)

- Participants reconvene and share insights and findings from each station.
- Discuss common themes, strengths and areas for improvement.
- Collaboratively prioritise action steps based on assessment results.

ACTION PLANNING AND COMMUNICATION (30 MINUTES)

- Teams develop action plans based on assessment findings, assigning responsibilities and setting timelines.
- Create posters or newsletter content to communicate progress, outcomes and action plans to team members.

CONCLUSION: COMMITMENT TO FLOURISHING (30 MINUTES)

- Participants reflect on the importance of ongoing assessment and commitment to development.
- Closing remarks and encouragement to continue the journey towards flourishing.

EXAMPLE OUTCOME

Following the 'Flourish-O-Meter' activity, staff and teams at your educational institution have engaged in a collaborative assessment process. They have gathered valuable insights from multiple sources, including peer feedback, turnover data, learner outcomes, stakeholder feedback, learner feedback, process evaluation and recruitment data.

Through discussion and action planning, they have identified areas for improvement and developed actionable strategies to enhance staff and team development. Visual posters and newsletter content have been created to transparently communicate progress, outcomes and action plans.

This activity catalyses continuous improvement and a commitment to flourishing within the institution. Staff members are aligned to create a positive learning environment where learners' needs are met and the institution's performance is consistently evaluated and enhanced.

ACTIVITY 7.11

Action-oriented Staff Meeting

An action-oriented staff meeting is useful for sharing and reviewing data and collaboratively identifying improvement actions. In planning for such a meeting, ensure staff have sufficient time to review the data and consider how the values underpinning the person-centred curriculum are reflected.

- You could start by revisiting the team's core values and shared objectives and clarifying the group task.
- Allow quiet time to review key metrics and data and ask team members to jot down their initial thoughts.
- Post-it notes can be used to capture thoughts and collate topics.
- Broad themes can be identified, and staff teams can be invited to work out solutions and actions to address the issues identified.
- Allow time for discussion and consensus opinion to be sought.

Promoting Robust Teams Where Everyone Belongs

It is also important to embed celebration and maintain a positive attitude, acknowledge and communicate progress, and commemorate the accomplishments of all staff and learners. Recognition of personal and collective achievements is essential in pursuing person-centred staff development. This process requires continuous effort to adhere to your vision (Figure 7.1) and constantly assess and improve collaboration with fellow team members. It would help if you did not wait until the completion of a project, exam, course or curriculum but use this throughout the entire curriculum developmental process.

This notion can be likened to the path depicted in Figure 7.1, which extends around the bend and stretches upward towards an unseen and far away goal. Although this may initially appear discouraging, it is crucial to view curriculum development as a way of life and a collaborative effort to enhance the well-being of all learners and staff. Sharing and commemorating positive experiences and accomplishments encountered along the journey are imperative to sustain our enthusiasm and drive. Acknowledging that becoming a person-centred staff member is a continuous process, embracing an inclusive approach is important, where individuals feel that they are genuine collaborators actively involved as valuable team members (Dewing et al. 2014). Further, recognising and celebrating accomplishments are vital in nurturing our motivation to engage and exert additional effort actively. It boosts energy when someone acknowledges our achievements and openly shares these accolades within the workplace.

Reflecting on your own experiences, it is worth pondering when you last exhibited or took part in affirmations of the achievements of others, expressing them out loud to both the individuals involved and their colleagues.

One way to get started could be 'champagne lunches' or 'award lunches', where a monthly lunch meeting is used to celebrate and share that month's achievement. This could be a publication, funding, an award, media coverage, course evaluation or

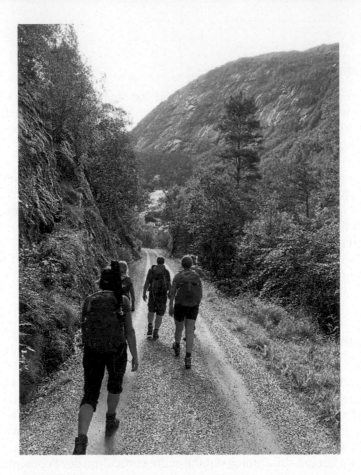

FIGURE 7.1   The pathway of curriculum development. *Source*: © H.K. Falkenberg.

birthdays. The list is endless. Of course, it does not need to be an award, but a celebratory event that values achievements within the team. One simple activity to get you started is to think about what your team members could be acknowledged for. This activity can be performed individually or as a team activity.

ACTIVITY 7.12

Reward and Recognition

Imagine you have three recognition awards to offer this week – who would you award them to, and for what reason? Imagine you could receive three awards – what would you receive them for?

Giving staff members 10 minutes to prepare this in advance is useful as a team activity. During the award lunch, ask staff to share who they would award. You should ensure that all staff are awarded for something within the first award lunches. If staff also share their thoughts on what they could be awarded for, it points towards the team being a safe space fostering a culture of sharing. In a person-centred culture, we are dedicated to providing sincere compliments and positive recognition of person-centredness in action or collaborating with a colleague who embodies person-centred values in their work ethos. Recognising the work of all team members should be encouraged and can be offered in general terms such as saying thank you or acknowledgement of support such as:

- Thank you for the work you did today.
- Thank you. I enjoyed working with you today.
- I wanted you to know that I admired how you responded with X today.
- I've learned a lot from observing your work this week.
- I appreciated your support today.
- I saw how helpful you were in supporting X, who was so busy.

Or in more specific terms:

- I saw that you facilitated the project group session well today. I felt you made sure that we were all clear about the purpose of the session and what we wanted to achieve at the beginning. You kept us on track in the middle by using the agenda, but you did not drag us through it. I also felt that you ensured that we had to contribute to group decisions about keeping on track. Great! I am learning to facilitate a session or meeting from watching you!

In the activities described above, you may find that it was much easier for you and your team to acknowledge a colleague's accomplishments than to share your own. In many work cultures, it is quite common to find it challenging to share accomplishments. This may be because we often are embarrassed to tell others what we have done well as we fear being perceived as self promoting or boastful, or believe our accomplishments are insufficient to interest others, or because the team culture leads to a collective avoidance of sharing one's achievements. The following activity, adapted from Dewing et al. (2014), facilitates sharing individual accomplishments and encourages mutual sharing among staff.

ACTIVITY 7.13

Share Achievements and Celebrate in a Team

This activity aims to facilitate you, in collaboration with your peers, such as your colleagues, active learning groups, team members or other relevant stakeholders, to contemplate how your accomplishments can be shared and celebrated in a learning environment. The activity may be conducted within an educational

(continued)

(continued)

context, such as an active learning group session, a team or staff meeting or the executive board. Alternatively, it may be carried out during a practice development session, such as a stakeholder group, project group, patients/students forum or social activity. Before you begin, check out what methods your organisation already uses.

One example is starting meetings with 'our recent accomplishments and/or things to celebrate'. This helps build commitment and resilience for the challenges to be discussed in the meeting. If you want to try something new, consider this activity which takes about 30 minutes. You will need:

- reflections on identifying, sharing and acknowledging own accomplishments (prepared in advance)
- post-it notes
- picture cards (face down)
- flipchart/whiteboard/display screen and pens
- one person to take the role of facilitator to structure the session and take summary notes.

Ask everyone to write their accomplishments on individual post-it notes. If anyone needs help, the facilitator will pair them with another team member who can help (5 minutes).

Ask people to arrange their sticky notes and organise them based on similarities, assigning a name (descriptor) to each theme (5 minutes).

Encourage people to provide positive feedback to one another (5 minutes).

Moving forward, everyone is asked to consider how they can share and celebrate these achievements. To stimulate this thinking process, the facilitator instructs them to randomly choose three picture cards (or five if working in pairs) and display them together face-up (5 minutes).

Taking individual pictures and the collection as a whole, participants are asked to share their ideas on how the team could share and celebrate the identified achievements. The aim is for people to voice their ideas spontaneously without overthinking. The facilitator will summarise these ideas on the flipchart/board (10 minutes).

Participants are guided to assess whether these impromptu ideas are worth pursuing or what steps need to be taken if they are not. The group is then prompted to agree on the first step and assign responsibilities for who will complete the necessary actions and by when. The facilitator will provide a record shortly after the session.

These activities can facilitate the sharing and celebrating of various accomplishments among the staff, learners and the team.

SUMMARY

- In this chapter, we have addressed the staff component of the Person-centred Curriculum Framework and the general attributes and qualities of the team needed to enable the facilitation of a person-centred learning culture.
- Individual and team support is critical in this context, where a continuous development of 'self' is required to design, deliver and sustain a person-centred curriculum where all learners flourish.

REFERENCES

Barnett, R. and Coate, K. (2005). *Engaging the Curriculum in Higher Education*. Buckingham: Open University Press.

Buchanan, D., Boddy, D., and McCalman, J. (2013). Getting in, getting on, getting out and getting back. In: *Doing Research in Organisations* (ed. A. Bryman), 53–67. Abingdon: Routledge.

Cardiff, S., McCormack, B., and McCance, T. (2018). Person-centred leadership: a relational approach to leadership derived through action research. *Journal of Clinical Nursing* 27 (15–16): 3056–3069.

Cowan, J., George, J.W., and Pinheiro-Torres, A. (2004). Alignment of developments in higher education. *Higher Education* 48: 439–459.

Dewing, J., McCormack, B., and Titchen, A. (2014). *Practice Development Workbook for Nursing, Health and Social Care Teams*. Chichester: Wiley.

Dickson, C., van Lieshout, F., Kmetec, S. et al. (2020). Developing philosophical and pedagogical principles for a pan-European person-centred curriculum framework. *International Practice Development Journal* 10 (Suppl 2): 1–20.

Hardiman, M. and Dewing, J. (2014). Critical ally and critical friend: stepping stones to facilitating practice development. *International Practice Development Journal* 4 (1): 3.

Jacobs, G. and Janssen, B. (2018). Eigen regie en waardigheid in de zorg: een kwestie van persoonsgerichte praktijkvoering. *Journal of Social Intervention: Theory and Practice* 27 (6): 48–64.

Lalleman, P., Bouma, J., Smid, G. et al. (2017). Peer-to-peer shadowing as a technique for the development of nurse middle managers clinical leadership: an explorative study. *Leadership in Health Services* 30 (4): 475–490.

Manley, K. and Jackson, C. (2019). Microsystems culture change: a refined theory for developing person-centred, safe and effective workplaces based on strategies that embed a safety culture. *International Practice Development Journal* 9 (2), article 4.

Masimula, Q.K., van der Wath, A.E., and Coetzee-Prinsloo, I. (2023). Implementing a program to transform the workplace culture towards person-centeredness in a public nursing education institution in South Africa. *International Journal of Africa Nursing Sciences* 18: 100541.

McCormack, B., McCance, T., and Martin, S. (2021). What is person-centredness? In: *Fundamentals of Person-centred Healthcare Practice* (ed. B. McCormack, T. McCance, and C.e.a. (e.) Bulley), 13–22. Oxford: Wiley.

Noben, I., Brouwer, J., Deinum, J.F., and Hofman, W.A. (2022). The development of university teachers' collaboration networks during a departmental professional development project. *Teaching and Teacher Education* 110: 103579.

O'Donnell, D., Slater, P., McCance, T. et al. (2021). The development and validation of the person-centred practice inventory-student instrument: a modified Delphi study. *Nurse Education Today* 100: 104826.

O'Donnell, D., Dickson, C., Phelan, A. et al. (2022). A mixed methods approach to the development of a person-centred curriculum framework: surfacing person-centred principles and practices. *International Practice Development Journal* 12 (Suppl 3): 1–14.

OECD (2022). *Education at a Glance 2022: OECD Indicators*. Paris: OECD Publishing.

Saroyan, A. and Trigwell, K. (2015). Higher education teachers' professional learning: process and outcome. *Studies in Educational Evaluation* 46: 92–101.

Titchen, A. (2004). Helping relationships for practice development: critical companionship. In: *Practice Development in Nursing* (ed. B. McCormack, K. Manley, and R. Garbett), 148–174. Oxford: Blackwell.

CHAPTER 8

Skills

In this chapter we aim to explore 'skills' in person-centred curricula and ways in which skills shape the way that the curriculum is positioned in programmes of work. We view skills as the actual knowledge, expertise and competence of educators, leaders or relevant others who are involved in developing and delivering the curriculum. This chapter focuses on the knowledge, expertise and skills needed by educators, and others, which collectively go towards creating the conditions and culture for all learners to flourish. Fundamentally, this is underpinned by the shared values of person-centredness. We will work with different attributes and core skills that offer methods, tools and approaches to bring these elements to life. We will connect with other sections of this book, for example, how skills and staff can merge to create conditions for person-centred learning and human flourishing, as well as skills and style in creating a healthful learning culture. The methods, tools and approaches we offer here are not exhaustive.

INTRODUCTION

This chapter focuses on the skills component of the Person-centred Curriculum Framework. In this framework, we define skills as:

> the actual knowledge, expertise, skills and competence of educators with responsibility for delivering and developing the curriculum.

We consider that those developing and delivering a person-centred curriculum should have the capabilities to collectively create the conditions for learners to flourish in a culture that is underpinned by the shared values of person-centredness (Cook et al. 2022, p. 6). This requires those involved in the curriculum (e.g. students, academics, practice colleagues supporting students, those in other education roles,

Developing Person-Centred Cultures in Healthcare Education and Practice: An Essential Guide, First Edition. Edited by Brendan McCormack.
© 2024 John Wiley & Sons Ltd. Published 2024 by John Wiley & Sons Ltd.

leaders and ambassadors) to have the necessary knowledge, skills and expertise to facilitate the delivery, development and/or evaluation of a person-centred curriculum. Attributes such as being professionally competent, having developed interpersonal skills, being committed to the job, being able to demonstrate clarity of beliefs and values, and knowing self, known as prerequisites in the person-centred practice framework, enable these professionals, as facilitators, to create healthful relationships with others. As such, these skills form partnerships of solidarity amongst those involved that lead to cultures of learning where students, and those supporting them, flourish.

In bringing facilitation skills to life, psychologically safe spaces for learning are forged and (critical, creative) dialogic relationships lead to the open sharing of thoughts, experiences and alternative ways of acting. Dialogic relationships of this kind are underpinned by principles of collaboration, participation, inclusion, respect, and individual and collective rights on autonomy and reciprocity. Dialogic relationships also recognise that knowledge and expertise are not fixed entities, but continually evolve as we are always in an unfinished state (Freire 1998). In the same respect, skills continually evolve as persons engaged in the curriculum grow into and from the curriculum, e.g. each interaction with a learner develops the educator as they develop students. In this respect, person-centred curricula are brought to life by the fusion of skills and values in a manner that is emancipatory in nature as it enlivens a critical consciousness, extending widely across the curriculum and the wider learning culture (Cook 2017).

Understanding who we are and who we are becoming necessitates an understanding of our relationship with the contexts we are part of and how to enable sustainable transformation for the better; this requires skilled facilitation. A person cannot fully understand that relationship from their singular perspective; they must be engaged in a critical dialogue with others to understand their views and those of others and the interplay between these views to construct a critical and shared informed view. This is complex, but illustrates the full attributes required of facilitators to create such conditions that support the delivery and development of a person-centred curriculum.

This relational and (mostly) dialogic encounter is underpinned by timely, transparent and practical feedback and feedforward but also necessitates a reflective and reflexive stance among all those involved that is informed by ongoing evaluation. Such a stance can be achieved in a number of ways but includes engaging with self and peer critique/ review that informs and engages investment in their knowledge, skills and expertise. In working dialogically, facilitators deploy their skills to create the conditions of learning that contribute to the creation/cultivation of a healthful culture whereby the shared values of person-centredness are brought to life and human flourishing can be experienced. The development and adoption of these skilled ways of working require a culture whereby persons are supported and encouraged to develop through continuous ways of learning that are critical, reflexive and collaborative (Cook 2017; Cook et al. 2022).

Facilitation is a way of working with others, through intentional use of self, using a set of skills used purposefully when working alongside another person, or with a group, enabling and supporting them to achieve their objectives, e.g. delivering and/or developing a person-centred curriculum.

The Learner-Educator-Experience Nexus

We consider learners to be those whom we teach, but they are also stakeholders and partners in the development of the programme.

Knowles (1975) historically identifies four key characteristics of the self-directed adult learner, in that they are self-directed, their past experiences enrich their learning, life experience influences motivation to learn, and they are inquisitive and self-motivated to learn. The educational approach therefore needs to be synergistic, whereby the learner is facilitated in their journey of identifying their learning needs, recognising the resources available to achieve learning and gaining the skills to evaluate their development. Such a facilitative approach recognises that knowledge is not given, it is developed through the learner-teacher (or facilitator)-experience nexus (Cook 2017). With learners not being a homogenous group, facilitation skills therefore need to be adaptable and flexible to the diversity of learners in a manner that is inclusive, regardless of where that learning environment is located. Teaching or education, in a form of transmission of knowledge, is limited. Rather, the skills required necessitate the facilitator to take a dynamic, developmental approach that centres on the individual or a group as the subject of learning and teacher or facilitator as mediator of the process; it is a praxis predicated upon dialogic relationships.

However, we need to consider facilitation that is more than a set of technical skills that promote discussion or facilitate dialogic engagement alone. As facilitation is a participative and integrated approach to learning, development and improvement in the workplace, a mix of skills is required – skills that enable relational connectedness, critical and creative dialogues and transformation. Regmi (2012) clarifies that to be an effective facilitator requires the person to be emotionally intelligent alongside an awareness of the power dynamic between the learner and facilitator. This requires reflection and reflexivity skills.

Reflexivity and reflection are related concepts but they have distinct characteristics. While both reflection and reflexivity involve introspection and learning from experiences, reflexivity goes further by emphasising the critical examination of one's own assumptions and their impact on designing and delivering a person-centred curriculum. It promotes a more nuanced understanding of the factors at play and encourages professionals to challenge their own perspectives to create more meaningful and equitable practices.

In deploying the skills of facilitation, it is more important to consider what this will lead the learner to do and learn, rather than focus on what the facilitator is doing. In person-centred curricula, though, striving for mutual learning and flourishing through feedback and feedforward is pivotal to this process.

Within our definition of skills, we identify that the knowledge, expertise, skills and competences needed by the academic team with responsibility for delivering the curriculum are synergistic with the other components of the framework and collectively these create the conditions for all learners to flourish in a culture underpinned by the shared values of person-centredness.

Arising from this, collaborators in the development of the Person-centred Curriculum Framework identified a range of thematic actions that should be considered when determining the skills that underpin a person-centred curriculum. These actions will shape the content of much of this chapter.

Thematic Actions

Develop skills to be a person-centred facilitator to enable a curriculum to be (come) person centred.

1. Being responsive to feedback and needs through individual and team practices.
2. Developing psychologically safe learning environments to create the conditions to be both challenging and supportive, and value individual personhood.
3. Creating person-centred environments for everyone to flourish.
4. Fostering relationships that are reciprocal, respectful, inclusive and collaborative.
5. Supporting or coaching learners in choosing their pathway in a flexible curriculum.

We therefore see skills as more than the things one does, also including the full attributes of those facilitating learning and transformation and how they use these attributes to deliver, support and develop a person-centred curriculum.

FREQUENTLY ASKED QUESTIONS ABOUT SKILLS

These questions are designed to help you consider what you have already as an individual or team, and what gaps exist in terms of delivering a person-centred curriculum. This analysis begins with understanding and agreeing shared values as a team; Chapter 5 provides a process for teams to begin this process and act as the first steps to understanding the team. From there, we explore the curriculum we want to have, the skills needed to deliver it and the skills gaps that may exist.

- How do you view skills in a person-centred curriculum?
- Why are skills important in person-centred curricula?
- What skills are necessary to deliver a person-centred healthcare curriculum?
- How would we know if our skills, as a team, are sufficient to deliver the curriculum?
- How could we improve or develop these skills?

UNPACKING THE STRATEGIC THEMES

Earlier, we identified the five strategic action themes that we synthesised from the many suggestions provided by project collaborators. Essentially, these themes facilitate the creation of a flourishing learning culture by deploying these skills in a relational, transformative manner. This moves the concept of skills forward from being static to living out the delivery and development of a person-centred curriculum, informing and being informed by the other parts of the Person-centred Curriculum Framework and guiding practice in a systematic way. Essentially these five themes can be summarised into the following areas of activity.

- Exploring skills needed to be a person-centred facilitator (in both delivering and developing contexts) and identifying skill gaps. This is necessary to support the delivery of a person-centred curriculum and for students to experience person-centred relationships (so they learn how to engage in person-centred care relationships).
- Celebrating team strengths.
- Developing and improving skills, individually and in groups/teams.
- Constructing safe learning spaces where people flourish through dialogic engagement, reciprocity, inclusivity and high challenge and support.
- Creating a system of support to maintain skilled facilitation.

In this section we unpack these strategic action themes and provide processes, tools and methods that can help you bring your curriculum delivery skills to life.

Facilitation

Facilitation is a practice that could be performed by anyone in the organisation whatever their function or position – leaders, educators, students, curriculum developers or a community of person-centred ambassadors who collectively lead the curriculum into the future (Cook et al. 2022). These individuals or groups could promote understanding and living to the values around person-centredness (role-modelling), instigate (co-) facilitation of curriculum development and strive for sustainable transformation.

Facilitation is a way of working with others, through intentional use of self, purposefully using a set of skills when working alongside another person or with a group; enabling and supporting them to achieve their objectives, e.g. designing or delivering a person-centred curriculum. This set of skills includes those that enhance relational connectedness such as enabling dialogues, criticality, creativity, empathy, flexibility, political astuteness as well as understanding diverse learning styles, assessing individual needs, adapting content to different abilities and fostering self-directed learning.

ACTIVITY 8.1

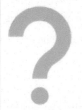

Think about your approach to education and ask yourself the following questions.

1. Do I facilitate learning as opposed to taking a didactic approach to education?
2. What facilitation skills am I confident in and which do I feel I need to develop?

It is important to know what facilitation means to you and what you are facilitating in a person-centred way. Knowing self as a facilitator and how this role is, or could be, part of your professional identity is critical to the practice of facilitation. Being clear about your intention as a facilitator helps create the conditions and culture for all learners to flourish in delivering and designing a person-centred curriculum.

Deciding on an Appropriate Strategy

Deciding on an appropriate facilitation strategy depends on what you want to use it for (its purpose), the context (what are they used to) and the person who is facilitating it (what you are good at). The circle of Sinek (2009) (Figure 8.1) could help guide this process. Purposes could vary from exploring existing knowledge, exploring practice, exploring new possibilities, testing and evaluation of actions, to analysing and/or making sense of what happens, etc. Strategies could also vary and be drawn from dialogical, creative, critical and research approaches. The overview of these strategies is unlimited, as new methods can always be found or created and new combinations of strategies could be initiated. Sometimes these strategies may already have a positive impact on the development process. The set-up of these strategies depends on the available time, means, space, people, material, etc. However, knowing the context and culture as a facilitator is necessary as this affects the impact of strategies on interpersonal processes. Sometimes this requires changing a structure, splitting up strategies, only using one aspect of a method, etc. It is important that this is a deliberate decision by you as a facilitator or as a group of facilitators.

Enabling Participation

Inviting others to participate in developing, designing and evaluating a curriculum is pivotal for all voices to be heard, to work with different ways of knowing as well as develop ownership of a sustainable person-centred curriculum. Doing a stakeholder analysis is important during the process. There are multiple sources available to help with this process. Table 8.1 provides a template that could be helpful in developing a communication plan with stakeholders.

In order to create safe and brave dialogical spaces for a healthful learning culture, constant attention needs to be given to the building and sustaining of (new) relationships. Because participation and collaboration in these processes are never static and

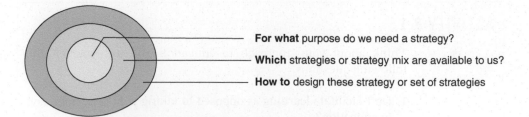

FIGURE 8.1 Adjusted circle of Sinek (2009) for strategy planning for facilitation.

TABLE 8.1 Stakeholder Analysis Template.

Who are your stakeholders?	How best to do this?	Who will communicate?
Those we will work with directly (these people might become members of the facilitation or ambassador group) Those you will consult Those you will inform		

the argument for and amount of participation could vary, activities for check-in and enhancing engagement and commitment should be ongoing areas of focus in developing group effectiveness.

ACTIVITY 8.2

Check-in

Before starting a meeting or a one-on-one conversation, you can decide to do this check-in activity. This helps to create safety first, to create an open space in which everyone can say what is important to them and their voice is heard.

Some 'rules' for check-in.

- It should be methodological; focus on the purpose of the being-together, possibly starting with a short contemplation activity.
- Start with a clear check-in question.
- Role model as a facilitator; it's okay to start with sharing your answer first.
- Be clear about the time you have for this activity; this creates a shared responsibility for timing.
- Popcorn-style: 'pop when you are hot, don't wait too long until you burn'; anyone who wants to say something can say it out loud, you don't need to wait for your turn.
- Sharing and dumping; don't react on each other's input.
- Summarise what has been said in the group, not on a personal level but rather to take it on a higher level. Everything that has been said is okay, and everything is a bit of everybody.

Some example questions for check-in.

- What have you been working on this week?
- What takes up most of your time?
- What milestones have you hit, in a work or private situation?
- What's in your way to being more person centred?
- What excites you about your work/private life?
- Or on a more light-hearted note: What book/person/film changed your worldview the most?

The hopes, fears and expectation activity is an effective way to gauge participants' attitudes about a project, workshop or any other collaborative engagement. It takes the tension and uncertainty out of a project by putting everything out in the open right from the start. It also gives each stakeholder time to voice and discuss what's most important to them as the project moves forward. When you see your concerns echoed by other team members, this creates a sense of camaraderie and group spirit – but it also triggers you to mitigate against these risks, as much as you can. At the same time, hearing everyone's ambitions and aspirations can be very motivating indeed. 'Hopes' reveal your teams' hopes about what can be accomplished. 'Fears' reveal their doubts about making an investment to work together. 'Expectations' reveal beliefs about what can be achieved in the reality of this kind of work and takes the specific context into account. It is typically completed as a group, helping to create empathy and shared excitement for new projects, workshops or other undertakings. During the activity, those participating take a moment to voice their hopes, fears and expectations and afterwards, the group discusses the points that have been raised with one another.

ACTIVITY 8.3

Hopes, Fears, Expectations

We've broken down the activity into a step-by-step process that you and your team can easily follow.

 ### STEP 1: EXPLAIN THE EXERCISE TO YOUR GROUP

First, you'll need to make sure that your group understands what you're doing and why. This gets everyone on the same page – knowing what to expect.

The hopes, fears and expectations exercise works best when everyone is open and honest. Participants should know that their contributions will be shared and then discussed. Wherever possible, avoid anonymity.

 ### STEP 2: EVERYONE WRITES DOWN THEIR HOPES, FEARS AND EXPECTATIONS

Hopes: What is each person looking forward to? What do they want to accomplish?

Fears: 'Fears' are situations team members want to avoid, issues they've had in the past, and what (if anything) they're cautious about moving forward.

Expectations: What is each person's expectation about their individual and collaborative achievement?

Next, pass out sticky notes or index cards for everyone to write down their hopes, fears and expectations. Each note should feature just one hope or fear or expectation – although there's no limit to how many sticky notes each person can have! It might be a good idea to offer some prompts to your team members, as this can fast-track the group to meaningful insights. Here are a few to get you started.

- I hope...
- I want to avoid...
- I'm worried about...
- I would love it if ...
- Last time [this happened] and that was great/not so great...
- For me, success looks like...

 ## STEP 3: POST EVERYONE'S HOPES, FEARS AND EXPECTATIONS ON LARGE SHEETS AND CREATE A VIEWING GALLERY

Before the meeting starts or while everyone is writing down their hopes, fears and expectations, you can use opaque tape to create a place on the wall for members to stick their notes.

Make sure the three sections are clearly separated but physically close enough to one another that you can discuss them in tandem. Once everyone has finished writing their notes, they should stick them to the wall.

 ## STEP 4: DISCUSS!

With everyone's hopes, fears and expectations up on the wall, it's time to discuss what your team members have to say.

Get each participant to point out their hopes, fears, expectations and elaborate on them a bit. Then ask other members to weigh in, before moving on to the next person. In total, this process should take anywhere from 30 to 45 minutes.

When discussing each person's input, make sure to address the cause or root of each point – and the likelihood of each hope, fear and expectation being realised. Try to find clusters in the contributions as this will create focus and ease the discussion. Try to come up with solutions to the fears and see if there are any correlating points between them and the hopes and expectations.

In addition, you can keep the sticky notes and can reflect on them during the process or at the end. You can ask each person to go back to their sticky note and write on the back what they might think about that hope, fear or expectation now and you can redo this activity again.

Exploring Your Desired Curriculum

One of the action themes is about exploring what curriculum you want to have. Therefore, activities on goal setting and visualising a common picture about what you want to achieve could support you in the process.

ACTIVITY 8.4

Visioning with Appreciative Inquiry

Appreciative inquiry (AI) is the skill of asking relevant and positive questions that promote individual and organisational strength. AI is collaborative and impacts several areas of functioning, including education. AI is about seeking the best in people – in the way they work, live and behave. The contemporary concept of AI came into focus after the article by David Cooperrider and Suresh Srivastava in 1987, in which they suggested that problem solving is 'overused' in organisational contexts and that active enquiries would perhaps be more helpful in creating innovations and ideas in the industry.

Using Appreciative Inquiry: the 5D Approach

1. 'Define' the Problem. Before you can analyse a situation, you need to define what it is you are looking at.
2. 'Discovery' Phase. Here you need to look for the best of what has happened in the past, and what is currently working well.
3. 'Dream' Phase. Here you imagine what could be. Dream about new possibilities. There are no restrictions placed on the potential of everyone's dream.
4. 'Design' Phase. Design brings together stories from discovery with the creative ideas from the dream phase. It is the phase where we bring together the best of what we have (discovery), with our imaginations of what might be (dream) to create what should be done – our ideal design plan.
5. 'Deliver' Phase. In this phase we create an action plan for implementing our ideal design plan.

Appreciative Inquiry: Guide for Workshop Facilitators – The Big Bang Partnership
    This visioning activity could be followed up by visioning the development process and developing ground rules. This is an activity you can do as a facilitator with a small informal group after a shared vision has been agreed.
    Examples of ground rules.

- Respect each other as people and co-workers and the different values, beliefs and views you all may hold.
- Listen to each other actively and do not talk over each other.
- Don't blame each other or others for when things go wrong but look for why they went wrong and plan together how to put them right.
- Offer each other high challenge and high support.
- Give each other honest feedback as a learning opportunity.
- Receive feedback non-defensively.
- Maintain confidentiality about what you tell each other unless you each agree otherwise.
- Carry out the actions you agree/commit to.
- Share out the responsibilities the group or team takes on in the future, e.g. take turns with organising meetings, taking notes, or sharing the actions to be carried out.

Reflexivity and Reflection

Reflexivity and reflection are related concepts but they have distinct characteristics, especially in the context of curriculum development and delivery.

Reflection refers to the process of looking back on one's experiences, actions and decisions to gain insights, learn from them and make improvements. It involves thoughtful consideration of what happened, why it happened and what can be learned from the experience. Reflection often involves analysing events and outcomes to identify strengths, weaknesses and areas for growth. It is a valuable tool for professionals to enhance their understanding, refine their skills and make informed decisions in their practice.

Reflexivity goes beyond reflection. It involves a deeper level of self-awareness and critical examination of one's own assumptions, biases and perspectives that influence actions and decisions. Reflexivity acknowledges that our thoughts and actions are shaped by our cultural, social and personal contexts. It encourages professionals to question their own beliefs, question power dynamics and consider the broader implications of their work. Reflexivity is about recognising how our own subjectivity affects the way we perceive and engage with the world, and it often leads to more transformative learning and growth.

In the context of developing practice, reflexivity involves being aware of and critically analysing the underlying values, assumptions and power dynamics that inform the development and implementation of new practices. It encourages professionals to question why certain practices are chosen, who benefits from them and who might be marginalised by them. Reflexivity leads to a deeper understanding of the complexities involved in developing practice and promotes a more inclusive, ethical and effective approach.

In summary, while both reflection and reflexivity involve introspection and learning from experiences, reflexivity goes further by emphasising the critical examination of one's own assumptions and their impact on designing and delivering a person-centred curriculum. It promotes a more nuanced understanding of the factors at play and encourages professionals to challenge their own perspectives to create more meaningful and equitable practices.

How to Engage Learners in Being Critical

Dewing (2008) stresses the importance of 'active learning' for achieving transformation in workplace cultures. She describes active learning as 'critical reflection, dialogue with self and others and engaging in learning activities in the workplace that make use of all our senses, multiple intelligences and doing things (i.e. workplace learning activities) together with colleagues and others' (p. 273). Dewing (2008, p. 274) emphasises 'that the more engaging an active the learning is, the more effective it is'. In active learning, enabling questions are pivotal. These are questions that will help us become more independent and effective learners. This is because they help us go further in the way we think or feel. We can then use new understandings to develop the curriculum to become more person centred. Enabling questions will help you to learn things for yourself rather than being dependent on others to tell you what to do or for advice.

Using enabling questions in our daily interactions with others as well as in active learning sessions will contribute to creating person-centred learning environments in education.

Enabling questions encourage reflection and can lead to action. They are open questions in that they do not make any assumptions.

Enabling questions examples.

- How do you feel about what happened?
- What could you do...?
- It sounds as though you are feeling... Tell me more about it.
- What do you think is really going on here?
- What does... mean to you?
- How can you...?
- How helpful was that comment?
- What question does that raise for you?
- How can we help you (or someone else) move forward on this issue?
- Perhaps it would be more helpful to turn that comment into a question.

Reflection and evaluation are different processes that could inform one and another. In the following section we provide an evaluation strategy that could be used in all kinds of different ways.

ACTIVITY 8.5

Claims, Concerns and Issues

Claims, concerns and issues (CCIs) is a really useful way in which you can gain the views and perspectives of all the people (stakeholders) who will be involved in and/or affected (in a positive or negative way) by the work you are planning to undertake. You can use it to explore any aspect of practice, e.g. timetables, assessment strategies etc., or to gain a sense of how a team are feeling – what they think is working well and what they would like to improve.

CCIs comes from Fourth Generation Evaluation (Guba and Lincoln 1989), an evaluation methodology that captures the opinions of stakeholders and uses these to plan ongoing activity.

A *claim* is a positive statement that someone would make about the subject, for example 'I believe feedback is important to help me to continuously develop my role within the team'.

A *concern* is a negative statement that someone would make about the same subject. 'I feel that there is a lack of positive and negative feedback for staff within the team both individually and as a group.'

An *issue* is a reasonable question about the subject; these are raised through a better understanding of the claims and concerns. What knowledge and skills do we need to develop to give and receive feedback effectively? How can we create opportunities to give feedback to each other?

For more information on facilitating a CCI exercise, visit the following site: www.fons.org/resources/documents/Creating-Caring-Cultures/CCIs.pdf

Use of Playfulness and Creative Approaches in Facilitation

Playfulness and creative approaches are not very common in higher education systems. Learning strategies are often rational and tend to overlook the emotional, affective and unconscious aspects of learning, and barriers to transformation. Instead, creative and arts-based approaches can be used to reveal these underlying issues. By uncovering tacit knowledge that would otherwise remain hidden, and revealing ways of being that would otherwise remain unexamined, opportunities for action can be increased. Such approaches are valuable for those engaged in taking action as they work towards lasting practice change. They stimulate the learner's formation of critical thinking, professional judgement and competence to act ethically in complex situations. There is a need for language, concepts, symbols and metaphors to understand the reality in which we work. It is important for learners to have the capacity for wondering and relate to that which is colourful, tone-rich, intangible and enigmatic.

In line with playful and creative approaches, the use of technology and digital capabilities should not be underestimated. This requires facilitators to be adaptive to technologies and digital capabilities and how these impact on our pedagogy and working with others. An example of a digital platform for collaborative work in an effective way is Mural. This platform helps to set up a variety of creative activities, from 'mind mapping sessions' to 'sprint planning'. It is far more than a whiteboard. You can use digital post-its, graphics and even pre-created formats to collaborate and collect input.

ACTIVITY 8.6

The Use of Metaphors

Metaphors are a creative and playful way of thinking and enlarge our frame of reference as they convey a message through the hidden connection between something familiar and something unfamiliar that goes beyond the literal meaning. Metaphors are a strong tool for sharing meaning and knowledge. They can contribute to clarifying what we see and hear and can give an extended meaning. As the essence of the metaphor is to understand an experience based on another, it is possible to lift one part of an experience and make it meaningful in a specific context.

Another example is the use of photo or picture cards that can support the finding of words to describe something that could be perceived as embodied knowledge and often hard to articulate.

Find Your System of Support

It is essential for facilitators, in particular those new to facilitation, to create a system of support to help to understand the characteristics of the context in which the curriculum has been developed and delivered. This is necessary to create balance in facilitation that is acceptable both to oneself and the context and which can then achieve synchronous working with learners.

Principles for action for facilitators that are assumed to contribute to the development of expertise for those engaged in the facilitation of a person-centred curriculum are as follows (van Lieshout 2013).

- Get to know yourself, your philosophical stance and transferable skills, both personal and professional. Get to know your supporters as people and explore and understand the educational practice context in all its dynamics.
- Develop a professional learning plan and discuss necessary support with your supporters. Pay attention to developing your ways of thinking, multiple knowing and intelligences and creative imagination.
- Decide on how to systematically record 'data' for reflection. Share your thoughts and feelings of imbalance and be open and honest about personal values and beliefs. Identify principles both espoused and in practice.
- Decide on actions that are most authentic in the relationship between the context and the supporters. Organise peer support, including for role modelling.
- Adopt a genuine approach to your whole self, appreciate yourself and have faith in yourself.
- Make time regularly for reflection on the development process as well as on process for support. Protect this time. Make use of all available sources of knowledge.

Together with the critical companionship model, the models of 'critical friend' and 'critical ally' offer a theoretically coherent framework for developing expertise in the facilitation of learning about practice from within the workplace. For more information see: www.fons.org/library/journal/volume4-issue1/article3

How Do You Know Facilitation Skills are Sufficiently Present and Available And/Or Whether There are Any Skill Gaps?

Facilitators can assess their skills for designing and delivering a person-centred curriculum by engaging in self-reflection and seeking feedback from colleagues, mentors and learners. They can attend workshops, courses and conferences related to curriculum development and person-centred approaches. Additionally, practising these skills in real-world settings and evaluating the outcomes can help professionals gauge their proficiency. Online resources, self-assessment tools and peer collaboration can also aid in identifying areas for improvement and continuous growth.

Combining different tools could lead to a more holistic exploration of the skills of professionals and teams and whether there is a gap that needs to be overcome. Several tools and methods can be relevant for assessing or measuring the skills required for designing and delivering a person-centred curriculum. The Person-centred Curriculum

Framework could be used to develop evaluation criteria that outline the specific skills required for designing and delivering a person-centred curriculum in your context and then can help you and your colleagues self-assess and receive feedback from peers or supervisors.

ACTIVITY 8.7

Where are We at?

This activity could be done individually or as group and needs to be orientated around the facilitation of developing, delivering or evaluating a person-centred curriculum. Its purpose is to identify positive and negative factors in the team that you can build on or address. The activity below is a different way of doing a SWOT analysis.

Each person takes a paper and pencils and puts their hand on the paper. You ask them to draw the contour of their hand. At each end you ask everyone to write down their answers on the questions below at each finger. You can collate all individual hands or draw one hand on a large whiteboard. You can explore and discuss the input as similar to the hopes, fears and expectation exercise.

Hand metaphor.

- Thumb: what are we as a department/team good at?
- Index finger: where are we going?
- Middle finger: what do we hate?
- Ring finger: what are we loyal to?
- Little finger: where is potential for growth for us?

Tools to Evaluate Our Delivery of Person-centred Education

The following may be useful in aiding evaluation of a team or the learner experience and can be used to inform where further development of the skills base may be needed.

- *Self-assessment surveys*: professionals can use self-assessment surveys or questionnaires specifically designed to evaluate their skills in curriculum development, such as their understanding of learning styles, adaptability and communication abilities.
- *Peer feedback*: engaging in peer observations and receiving constructive feedback from colleagues or mentors can provide valuable insights into one's strengths and areas that need improvement.

- *Portfolio review*: creating a portfolio showcasing examples of person-centred curriculum development projects, along with reflections on challenges faced and strategies used, can demonstrate proficiency to others and provide a basis for self-reflection.
- *Observations and reflections*: regularly observing and reflecting on how learners engage with the curriculum, as well as outcomes and adjustments made, can provide insights into the effectiveness of one's approach.
- *Feedback from learners*: collecting feedback directly from learners about their learning experiences, preferences and challenges can help professionals understand how well they are meeting individual needs.
- *360° feedback*: this form of feedback seeks anonymous responses from others to help build a picture of strengths and challenges to our approach to a variety of matters.

How are Skills Monitored and Improved?

Once we know what our baseline is, we need to consider how we can develop and continually improve the skills we have to provide a quality approach to a person-centred curriculum. There are several ways in which we can do this.

- *Professional development plans*: creating professional development plans (as individuals, teams or organisations) that outline goals, strategies and milestones for improving curriculum development skills can provide a structured approach to skill enhancement.
- *System of support – critical companionship*: having a mentor, critical friend or undertaking coaching can create a system of support that gives you a clear pathway to development, reviewing your progress at intervals.
- *Collaborative learning communities*: participating in collaborative learning communities, either online or in-person, can facilitate discussions, idea sharing and skill refinement through interactions with peers and experts. You could be the person to initiate a community of practice where it is needed, helping to develop yourself and others.
- *Courses (including online) and workshops*: enrolling in courses and workshops focused on curriculum development, person-centred approaches and related skills can offer structured learning and opportunities for skill assessment.

Remember that continuous self-assessment, active learning and seeking diverse sources of feedback, and affirming others, are crucial for professionals to enhance their skills in designing and delivering effective person-centred curricula (see Chapter 7).

Celebrating Team Strengths and Strategies for Enhancing These

A key skill to promote robust teams where all members feel they belong is the ability to value and celebrate team diversity. Strategies to promote authentic collaboration in all areas of curriculum development should be encouraged and become part of the team culture. Celebrating all achievements is not always ingrained within the workplace culture, and some team members may feel hesitant to share their accomplishments.

It is important to develop the necessary skills to facilitate sharing and provide positive recognition for these achievements.

To address this concern, we present some activities aimed at facilitating a deeper understanding of the purpose and potential impact of sharing and celebrating, as well as providing opportunities to acquire the necessary skills (Dewing et al. 2014). One tool to promote team strength is to celebrate all successes small and big on a regular basis, as described in Chapter 7.

Acknowledging Your Own Accomplishments

To develop the skills, it can be useful to consider acknowledging achievements in different levels.

- Acknowledging your own accomplishments.
- Affirming and acknowledging each other's accomplishments.
- Acknowledging and affirming everyday achievements.

The following activities are adapted from Dewing et al. (2014).

ACTIVITY 8.8

Do you acknowledge your achievements to yourself? If not, carrying out a personal creative visualisation exercise is one method to aid in this process. Alternatively, you can mentally revisit the accomplishment from its inception and contemplate your contributions towards the achieved successes.

You will need:

- 15 minutes
- a notebook
- a quiet space to reflect on your own.

Creative visualisation (5 minutes) – after you have read these instructions, close your eyes. Tell yourself that you have 15 minutes learning space entirely for yourself. Undertake the following steps.

- Take a few deep breaths. Feel the rise and fall of your chest. Hear the sound of your breath.
- Imagine your experience in the practice development as a river. In your imagination, take yourself back to the source of the river (the starting point of the practice development). Now make your way down the river, experiencing all the twists and turns, the rocks and rapids, the waterfalls and the quiet flows and pools. How do you see yourself, in your mind's eye, as you move down the practice development river?

(continued)

(continued)

- When you get to where you are now, gently open your eyes. Now reflect on the part you played and are playing now.
  - What did you do (are doing) to navigate rocks, rapids, waterfalls, quiet flows and pools?
  - What successes or achievements have come about from your contribution?
- Now make notes on your achievements. Let what you didn't do so well float away for now.

ACTIVITY 8.9

Take 10 minutes to think about the last 24 hours. Write down all the things that have happened to you that you feel grateful or happy for. You should aim to write at least five things down.

1.
2.
3.
4.
5.

You can also find some helpful web-based tools on how to cultivate gratitude or the ability to uplift others at https://hsq.dukehealth.org/tools

---

Affirm and Acknowledge Each Other's Accomplishments

As described in Chapter 7, sharing our own accomplishments and affirming others will help to foster a person-centred culture. However, many people find it difficult to share their own achievements. It is a skill to create a culture for the sharing of individual accomplishments and encourage mutual sharing among staff. The objective of this team activity is to promote sharing accomplishments with each other. It also serves as an opportunity to practise the enabling questions introduced earlier and receive additional feedback about our effectiveness.

ACTIVITY 8.10

This activity can be done with two team members, but it is better with a group of three people (presenter, helper and observer). The time required is approximately 60 minutes with three people or 40 minutes with two. You will need:

- to have done Activity 8.8 above in advance and written down reflections on your achievements

- a space somewhere in the public area of the workplace where you are not in the way, but where you can sit together and talk. You will be learning how to share and celebrate achievements in the space where curriculum development happens
- to explain to fellow colleagues and learners what you are doing and negotiate with them so that you will not be unduly interrupted.

If you are working in pairs, you will be an observer at the same time as a presenter or helper. The timing for each presentation is 15 minutes including acknowledging and affirming by the helper and five minutes for feedback.

PRESENTER

In the context of your work, share a personal or collective achievement that you have encountered. The achievement is to be shared with the designated helper; try being short and to the point. The achievement should be one that you are proud of and focus on the positive outcomes (10 minutes).

HELPER

As a helper, your role is to assist the presenter in critically analysing their achievement and understanding the specific factors that contributed to its success (within the 10 minutes). A tip is to ask the observer to inform you when 10 minutes have passed. Ask open-ended questions, such as 'How do you know?' and 'What does this mean?' to prompt the presenter's reflection. The aim is to guide the presenter in defining or redefining their achievement in precise detail and understanding their role in it. This will enable the presenter to reflect on the impact of their achievement on themselves and other learners/colleagues, and consider its implications for facilitating a sharing culture. Some potential guiding questions could include the following.

- It seems like you have some positive feelings related to this achievement. Could you elaborate on these feelings?
- How do you personally feel about this achievement?
- In your opinion, what factors contributed to its success?
- What specific actions did you take to contribute to this achievement?
- How have you managed to recognise and appreciate the value of your own accomplishment?
- In what ways can you share this achievement with others?

When the 10 minutes are up, the helper recognises the presenter's accomplishment, expresses gratitude for sharing and provides details of why it is considered an achievement. The helper should not focus on or unpick negative facets of the event or story. The aim lies in the ability to identify and value the success (5 minutes).

(continued)

(continued)

OBSERVER

The observer assumes an active listening role throughout the entire 15-minute duration, attentively processing the communication. The observer focuses on the presenter's ability to maintain a positive attitude and evaluates the effectiveness of the helper's different questions and responses in facilitating the presenter's ability to share and acknowledge their success. Additionally, the observer notes the impact of acknowledgement and appreciation on the presenter. The observer also pays attention to the emotions exhibited by both the presenter and the helper in relation to success.

Further, the observer assesses the level of investment demonstrated by the presenter in sharing the achievement. This includes evaluating the presenter's will, commitment and motivation to build upon the accomplishment and enhance a sharing workplace culture.

In addition, the observer may also wish to consider whether the helper effectively conveys genuine praise and affirmation.

- Is the helper conveying the praise and affirmation in a way that feels real?
- What is the effect of the acknowledgement and affirmation?
- Is the presenter focusing on the positive of what they have done and learned about?

Following the session and a brief pause, the presenter and helper share their individual experiences, with the presenter speaking first, followed by the helper, each given one minute to convey their thoughts. The observer finally provides feedback to the helper for five minutes, highlighting how their facilitation positively impacted the presenter. The observer also offers feedback to the presenter and the helper (five minutes). At this point, the presenter and helper may choose to share their own comments. To ensure equal participation, the roles of helper and presenter are then switched among the group members, allowing each person to experience each role.

Acknowledging and Affirming Everyday Achievements

Are you skilled in recognising and affirming the accomplishments of others? When someone performs well, do you informally show gratitude and give praise throughout the workday? Or is it also done formally and intentionally during regular staff/team meetings and learning development sessions? Is there a designated time or arena for sharing positive news? Particularly for team leaders or managers, do you try to acknowledge people's efforts when you can, in corridors, public spaces, meetings, staff development reviews and personal development planning?

Are you able to recognise when you have received praise, whether it is general or specific? Often, we are unable to do so. Consequently, we feel that we are never acknowledged or praised, when we simply cannot perceive it ourselves.

ACTIVITY 8.11

The aim of this individual activity is to:

- keep a log documenting when you acknowledge and affirm others throughout the work day (you can use the logbook template below)
- reflect upon the impact of providing acknowledgement and praise on the person, yourself and practice development
- recognise when you have received recognition and praise for your own efforts.

When doing this, you can include a wide variety of people you come into contact with daily.

The following template may be useful for both the learning log and reflection.

Logbook template

Acknowledgement (date and brief description)	Impact on person to whom given	Impact on you	Impact on person-centred workplace/ curriculum	Actions to be taken (what/by who/when)

Authentic Collaboration, Enhancing Diversity

Another way to promote person-centred skills development is to participate in inter-disciplinary courses/activities/networks. In our previous work with the person-centred curriculum, we developed a digital interdisciplinary doctoral supervision course. The course was equivalent to five ECTS and consisted of both independent self-learning and four facilitated webinars. The webinars were key to sharing experiences and learning how to develop as a person-centred supervisor, in an international environment. Learning together with other persons from a different scientific background and with a wide range of experience was very fruitful in promoting reflection upon individual skills in person-centred supervision of doctoral students. It also enabled the identification and acknowledgement of the importance of different points of views necessary at different stages, which are important transferrable skills in developing a team to enhance delivery of a person-centred curriculum.

This is how we advertised the course, as an example of how you can organise such a collaboration.

Online Course on Person-centred Doctoral Supervision (5 ECTS)

Are you supervising doctoral students or want to supervise doctoral students?
Do you want to enable your students to come into their own?
Do you also think this can be challenging and requires specific competencies?
Are you keen to learn from others and their approaches to supervision?

Why not come to this FREE online course and explore how to meet the challenges of being a supervisor in a person-centred way and join an international community?

We are running a seven-week pilot for a five ECTS independent self-directed learning experience course with four facilitated 60-minute online sessions on October 11 and 18 and November 1 and 22 2022, as part of an Erasmus+ project.

WHO SHOULD ATTEND THE COURSE?

Those that already supervise or are going to supervise doctoral students and who want to learn and develop their competencies in their engagement with students, supervisory team and other stakeholders, in and through an international community. Those who wish not only to guide doctoral students through the process but also to facilitate their learning and to learn from them too.

WHAT IS THE BACKGROUND TO THE COURSE?

In 2019, six partners from the UK, Ireland, The Netherlands, Norway and Slovenia began work on an Erasmus+ funded project to develop a curriculum framework that could support higher education and healthcare organisations in designing, delivering and evaluating the development of future person-centred healthcare practitioners. To ensure international relevance, the project adopted an evolutionary process, engaging multiple stakeholders from across each partner country at each stage. The aim of this school is to equip those leading healthcare curricula with the knowledge, skills and expertise to design, deliver and evaluate the education of future person-centred practitioners.

WHAT ARE THE INTENDED LEARNING OUTCOMES?

By the end of the seven-week course participants will be able to:

- articulate the philosophical, methodological and pedagogical principles underpinning person-centred doctoral supervision
- identify the conditions for creating safe spaces that support person-centred doctoral supervision
- develop person-centred practices in the delivery and evaluation of doctoral supervision.

WHAT WILL PARTICIPATION IN THE COURSE INCLUDE?

The course consists of independent self-learning in combination with four online facilitated modules held between October 2022 and November 2022. The first module is an introduction to the course, followed by three modules orientated around the three learning outcomes. The majority of work will be self-learning.

Each module requires some individual reading and/or collaborative work with participants prior to an interactive online session. The online sessions will be facilitated by members of the Erasmus+ team. CANVAS will be used as a shared learning environment.

The course will be closed with a reflective account around new insights you have gained from the course and thoughts on how to apply your new supervisory skills. To complete the course and to receive a certificate of attendance of five ECTS, you need to attend all the sessions, participate in the coursework and hand in the reflective account.

Seeking and Providing Feedback

You will have explored elements of seeking and providing feedback in Chapter 5 and, in this section, we are bringing you back to focus on aspects related to skills. Educators of a person-centred curriculum should be able to establish the conditions necessary for everyone to thrive in a culture that is based on the shared values of person-centredness. Self and peer critique is a tool educators can use to advance their knowledge, experience and skills (Gómez and Valdés 2019).

Actively seeking feedback from learners and peers about their experience of the curriculum is a skill that educators can develop and refine and when effective, it can be a powerful force for transformation (Dewing et al. 2014). The purpose of feedback is to challenge and support educators to see what they are doing well and the effect it has, as well as understanding how they can develop their knowledge and skills further.

Educators can use the following feedback cues to develop their skills of giving and actively seeking feedback, and how to respond to it so that it is nurturing and developmental. This can also form the basis of a discussion as to what feedback is and is not and what its purpose is.

Indicators of Effective Feedback (Dewing and Titchen 2007)

For the receiver

Acceptance	Indicates a willingness to accept feedback and listen actively (without talking). Receiver should only interject if the giver of the feedback is giving the feedback inappropriately.

(continued)

Active engagement	Listens carefully and tries to understand the meaning of the feedback.
	Interacts appropriately with the speaker, asking for clarification when needed.
	Gives an indication that action will be forthcoming. Considers what can be agreed with and anything that cannot be agreed with.
	Asks for further feedback on any areas for which feedback was needed but was not offered.
	Asks clarifying questions about things not understood.
	Decides what to do with the feedback – this may include seeking further feedback from others.
Authentic	Is genuine about wanting to listen, understand and take responsibility for owning feedback and doing something about it.
Open	Listens without frequent interruption or objections.
Reflective	Tries to understand the personal behaviour that has led to the feedback.
	Reflects at the time on feelings about the feedback.
Respectful	Recognises the value of what is being said and the speaker's right to say it without dismissing them.
Responsive	Willing to hear what's being said without turning the table on the giver of feedback.

For the giver

Supportive	Delivered in a non-threatening and encouraging manner for the receiver.
Direct	The focus of the feedback is clearly stated. The feedback is said clearly without deviation or repetition. The giver owns the feedback as coming from themselves. Feedback starts with 'I' and avoids 'everyone thinks'.
Sensitive	Delivered with sensitivity to the needs of the other person(s). Starts with the positive or a positive statement. Appreciation is offered to the other person where they have said they would like feedback. The giver, when talking about feelings the behaviour creates, does this with 'I feel ... angry/sad, etc.' not 'you make me feel ...'.
Considerate	Feedback is intended not to insult or demean and should be descriptive, not judgemental or evaluative – do not tell the other person why you feel they do something in a certain way.
Specific	Feedback is focused on specific behaviours or events and not general comments. Stick to one piece of feedback at a time. Where several pieces of feedback are needed, do not jump around or go back. Move forward.
Healthy timing	Given as close to the prompting event as possible and at an opportune time. The amount of time set aside for feedback is reasonable and not prolonged.

| Thoughtful | Well considered rather than impulsive – non-worked-through feelings or thoughts are held rather than blurted out. |
| Helpful | Feedback is intended to be of value to the other person and focuses on the behaviour of the person, not the person. |

Indicators of Ineffective Feedback (Dewing and Titchen 2007)

Attacking	The receiver verbally attacks the person giving feedback.
	The giver either gives inappropriate feedback (negative criticism) or gives feedback at the wrong time. They may use role or authority within the organisation as part of the above.
Closed	Declines opportunities to engage with feedback.
	Once in feedback situations, ignores the feedback or listens in a superficial way with little intention of processing and understanding the feedback.
Defensiveness	Objects to being given feedback.
	Defends own actions or reasons for actions.
Denial	Declines to accept the legitimacy of feedback.
	Often dismissive of feedback and of the person giving the feedback.
Lack of respect	Demonstrates devaluing of the person offering feedback or their right to speak by not listening, interrupting or talking over the person.
Passiveness	Makes little or no attempt to actively engage with the feedback or the feedback process or others involved.
Rationalisation	Offers detailed explanations for feedback that often show the receiver as having no responsibility or a poor level of self-awareness.
Superficial	Listens and agrees but does not engage with feedback. May avoid agreeing to actions or agrees with little intention of carrying them through.

Being responsive to feedback to create safe learning environments and the conditions for everyone to flourish

---

ACTIVITY 8.12

Think of times when you have been given feedback.

(continued)

(continued)

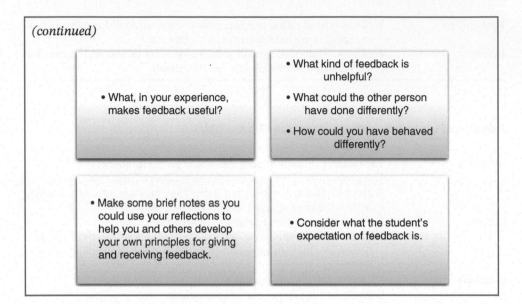

* What, in your experience, makes feedback useful?

* What kind of feedback is unhelpful?

* What could the other person have done differently?

* How could you have behaved differently?

* Make some brief notes as you could use your reflections to help you and others develop your own principles for giving and receiving feedback.

* Consider what the student's expectation of feedback is.

Looking After Self, Being Reflexive and Facilitation of Own Learning (Self as Active Learner)

Educators need to be continually aware of their own practice and development in order to keep the person-centred curriculum aligned to its underlying purpose and values. In Chapter 1 we acknowledge that it can be difficult for us to recognise that we might not be as person centred as we think we are and that we can have a 'blind spot' to our own way of being and doing. Individuals and relationships are continuously subjected to intrapersonal, interpersonal and contextual influences, so being a person-centred facilitator in everyday practice is no mean feat. Van Lieshout and Cardiff (2015) found that four principles help sustain balance in self and relational reciprocity while facilitating in a person-centred way:

1. being other-centred without losing self
2. valuing a constant state of becoming
3. maintaining relational connectedness
4. consciously working with context and cultures.

ACTIVITY 8.13

Reflective Space

This is a reflective activity that you can do on your own or with a colleague who poses the questions to you. The aim is to do this at a quick pace, so that you say things quickly and don't dwell on them too much. Your colleague writes down the key words you say.

• What values and beliefs do you still hold that no longer serve your learners well?

 • What new values and beliefs do you need to adopt?

 • What new beliefs or ideas do you need to put into action in order to improve your personal effectiveness?

 • How can you put the new ideas and belief structures into action in your daily life?

 • What will you read, study and learn that will help you become more person-centred?

 • What will you stop spending your time and energy on?

 • What three actions will you take to being more person-centred?

 • What changes will others notice in you?

 • What changes will others notice in your behaviours and your actions? Will the changes you make be enough for them to be visible to those around you? Are they significant enough to be noticed?

 • How will these changes impact on learners?

Maintaining Momentum

It is important to find ways to keep motivated and energised and adopt fresh approaches to curriculum delivery to create safe learning environments where everyone can flourish.

ACTIVITY 8.14

Keeping It Fresh Every Day

The purpose of this activity is to jump-start creativity when you find yourself and others becoming stale or falling into old ruts in your practice. At times when you have stopped being mindful or active in your learning, doing, being and becoming, it will help you to draw on your own (and others') resources to devise ways of keeping your practice fresh in your hearts and minds. Try to work with this guidance.

The activity can be done on your own, with your buddy or in a small, informal group (like an active learning group). You will need:

- approximately 30–45 minutes
- one of you to be facilitator if you are working in a group
- to establish ways of working
- a space to move around in
- personal notebook
- flipchart paper
- materials – felt-tip pens, paints, crayons, pastels, coloured paper or card (plus any other drawing materials you may want)
- a camera (e.g. on your phone).

This activity involves creating a short comic strip about transforming your practice from staleness to freshness.

If you are facilitating a group activity, explain the purpose and key activities and structure the session. You can take part as well, but you will need to keep an eye on the timings.

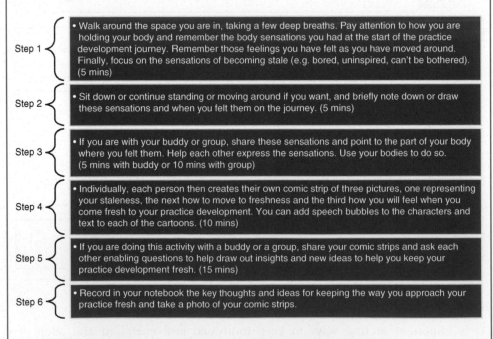

Step 1
- Walk around the space you are in, taking a few deep breaths. Pay attention to how you are holding your body and remember the body sensations you had at the start of the practice development journey. Remember those feelings you have felt as you have moved around. Finally, focus on the sensations of becoming stale (e.g. bored, uninspired, can't be bothered). (5 mins)

Step 2
- Sit down or continue standing or moving around if you want, and briefly note down or draw these sensations and when you felt them on the journey. (5 mins)

Step 3
- If you are with your buddy or group, share these sensations and point to the part of your body where you felt them. Help each other express the sensations. Use your bodies to do so. (5 mins with buddy or 10 mins with group)

Step 4
- Individually, each person then creates their own comic strip of three pictures, one representing your staleness, the next how to move to freshness and the third how you will feel when you come fresh to your practice development. You can add speech bubbles to the characters and text to each of the cartoons. (10 mins)

Step 5
- If you are doing this activity with a buddy or a group, share your comic strips and ask each other enabling questions to help draw out insights and new ideas to help you keep your practice development fresh. (15 mins)

Step 6
- Record in your notebook the key thoughts and ideas for keeping the way you approach your practice fresh and take a photo of your comic strips.

After the activity, you might like to reflect further on instances when you recognise that you were slipping back into old, non-person-centred ways or language using reflection. You might decide to share the comic strips with others involved in the curriculum to stimulate discussion about what they mean and thus alert others to the importance of keeping things fresh, or you may use it as a personal reminder.

Networking

Networking is an important arena for sharing and engaging others in person-centred curriculum development. The motivation for acquisition of knowledge and self-development can be enhanced through networking with peers in other person-centred healthcare curricula and with similar interests. Joining or having an affiliation with online knowledge networks can be a useful way to share knowledge and access expertise and resources. Networking is a way of engaging with others while developing relationships to provide support and enhance collaboration, inclusiveness and participation. Knowledge networks and communities of practice can be established in your organisation or across organisations regionally, nationally and internationally.

To get you started, spend 10 minutes identifying what network you are already engaged in. Ask yourself why you attend, what type of network it is and your role. Examples can be own workplace, local, regional, national or international, research, education, learning, student, emotional, practice, interdisciplinary, etc. Is there any network you want to become engaged with and how are you going to manage this? Answers here can be attending different types of meetings, conferences, dissemination, writing papers, social media, and inviting or initiating your own network. It is also important to have an emotional network (network of trust). Who are your closest confidants?

Network (individual persons/ other networks)	Type of network (learning/research/ clinical/emotional/ national/regional/ international)	Motivation to participate	What role do you have (initiator/ attender/ expert/ learner)?	Are changes needed (what/how/ when)?

SUMMARY

- In this chapter we have seen how skills are fundamental to bringing person-centred curricula to life.
- Skills are the tools of educational practice, embedded in active learning and development through the creation of dialogic, engaged learning environments where students learn, reflect and think critically as they develop the attributes of person-centred practitioners.

- The focus on skills in this chapter continues the processes you have seen from chapter to chapter in this book whereby collaborative, inclusive and participative approaches are embedded through the skills of the educator.
- Skills are aligned and synergistic with the principles of living out person-centred values and practices, role-modelling these within a person-centred culture.

REFERENCES

Cook, N. (2017). Co-creating Person-centred Learning and Development Experiences with Student Nurses in Practice through Action Research. Doctoral dissertation, Ulster University.

Cook, N.F., Brown, D., O'Donnell, D. et al. (2022). The person-centred curriculum framework: a universal curriculum framework for person-centred healthcare practitioner education. *International Practice Development Journal* 12 (4): 1–11.

Dewing, J. (2008). Chapter 15. Becoming and being active learners and creating active learning workplaces: the value of active learning. In: McCormack, B., Manley, K.,Wilson, V. (Eds.), International Practice Development in Nursing andHealthcare. Blackwell, Oxford, pp. 273–294.

Dewing, J. and Titchen, A. (2007). *Workplace Resources for Practice Development*. London: Royal College of Nursing.

Dewing, J., McCormack, B., and Titchen, A. (2014). *Practice Development Workbook for Nursing, Health and Social Care Teams*. Oxford: Wiley Blackwell.

Freire, P. (1998). *Pedagogy of Freedom: Ethics, Democracy, and Civic Courage*. Lanham: Rowman and Littlefield.

Gómez, L. and Valdés, M. (2019). The evaluation of teacher performance in higher education. *Purposes and Representations. Journal of Educational Psychology* 7 (2): 499–515.

Guba, EG and Lincoln, YS. (1989). Fourth Generation Evaluation. Newbury Park, Sage.

Knowles, M. (1975). *Self Directed Learning: A Guide for Learners and Teachers*. Chicago: Follet.

van Lieshout, F. (2013). Taking Action for Action. A study of the interplay between contextual and facilitator characteristics in developing an effective workplace culture in a Dutch hospital setting, through action research. PhD thesis, University of Ulster.

van Lieshout, F. and Cardiff, S. (2015). Reflections on being and becoming a person-centred facilitator. *International Practice Development Journal* 5 (Special issue): Article 4.

Regmi, K. (2012). A review of teaching methods – lecturing and facilitation in higher education (HE): a summary of the published evidence. *Journal of Effective Teaching* 12 (3): 61–76.

Sinek, S. (2009) Start with Why: How Great Leaders Inspire Everyone to Take Action. Brentford, Portfolio.

RESOURCES

Centre for Person-centred Practice Research: http://cpcpr.org

Duke Center for Healthcare Safety and Quality – well-being tools: https://hsq.dukehealth.org/tools

CHAPTER 9

Motivational Stories

In this final chapter, we present stories of person-centred developments undertaken by members of the Person-centred Curriculum (PCC) Framework project team and co-authors of this book. These stories illustrate both the processes of and outcomes from the implementation of person-centred learning and developments. They act as a means of integrating the different components of the 7S framework, bringing learning and development practices alive to the reader and inspiring similar developments. We don't present these stories as ideal practices or benchmarks of excellence in person-centred teaching, learning and assessment. Instead, we hope they give voice to different perspectives on bringing a person-centred lens to the curriculum in different contexts. The PCC Framework is presented as a holistic template for curriculum development but we recognise that in many situations, the starting point of curriculum development will be different and will incorporate some or all the development stages. Therefore, these stories highlight different parts of the framework and how learning for different purposes and contexts has been developed and implemented.

While the authors of these stories had the freedom to narrate their story in whatever way they wished, they were asked to follow a format as guidance in unfolding the details.

1. The focus of the story and the S it most links with
2. Where the story happened
3. Who were the key actors in the story
4. What they did
5. What worked
6. What didn't work/need further attention
7. What has been the key learning from this work
8. What next?

In Table 9.1 and Figure 9.1 we present a reminder of the 7S framework, upon which the PCC Framework is structured and with which each story in this chapter connects.

Developing Person-Centred Cultures in Healthcare Education and Practice: An Essential Guide, First Edition.
Edited by Brendan McCormack.
© 2024 John Wiley & Sons Ltd. Published 2024 by John Wiley & Sons Ltd.

TABLE 9.1 The 7S Framework with Definitions of Each Element.

Element	Definition
Strategy	This is the whole learning and development framework that identifies the unique selling point (USP) of the programme and what makes it unique, and thus attractive to potential stakeholders.
Structure	How the learning and development are structured (modules/units/courses) to achieve the intentions of the development activities as well as how the organisation/department is organised in terms of its structures to deliver the activities, including learner/stakeholder engagement and processes to meet the intended regulatory requirements and quality standards.
Systems	Teaching, learning, facilitation, assessment and evaluation methods used to achieve the stated development outcomes.
Shared values	The core values of the organisation/department and how these are made explicit in the person-centred developments.
Style	The style of leadership used to deliver the developments.
Staff	The general capabilities of the team with responsibility for delivering the developments, the skill mix of the team and the support for staff development to deliver the work, i.e. the make-up of the team, its 'fit' with the development intentions and staff support to deliver outcomes.
Skills	The actual knowledge, expertise, skills and competence of the academic team with responsibility for delivering the development processes and outcomes.

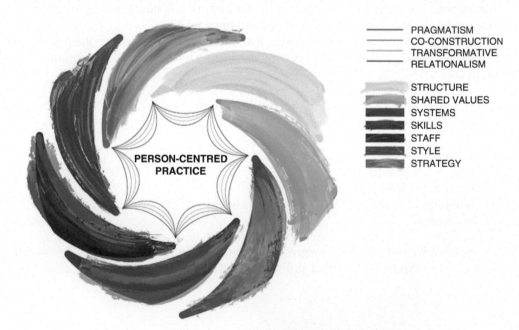

FIGURE 9.1 The 7S person-centred curriculum framework.

The stories are presented in a particular order, moving from a whole-system focus through to departmental developments and culture change and onwards to consider developments in leadership, knowledge and skills development and assessment.

STORY 1: THE POWER OF COLLABORATIVE WORKING – THE ULSTER UNIVERSITY STORY

Deirdre O'Donnell, Donna Brown, Neal Cook, Stephanie Dunleavy and Tanya McCance

This story details the experiences of colleagues at Ulster University and our partners, in progressing person-centredness in healthcare curricula since 2007. Our account demonstrates the whole team's sustained commitment to developing the healthcare workforce for person-centred practice. We work collaboratively to provide educational opportunities that advance knowledge and expertise in person-centred practice. This includes embedding person-centred philosophy and principles in undergraduate and postgraduate healthcare curricula, drawing upon our collective successes regionally, nationally and internationally in advancing academic practice in this field. This story embraces all the 7Ss but primarily highlights the centrality of shared values in harnessing the power of collaborative working.

Our team comprises the 170 staff that work in the School of Nursing and Paramedic Science at Ulster University in Northern Ireland. It also includes our partners who are academics, students, professionals with education roles across healthcare settings, and those holding strategic positions influencing healthcare curricula and workforce planning. Together, we support a diverse portfolio of 38 undergraduate and postgraduate person-centred healthcare programmes (14 of which are professionally regulated), across two campuses and via distance learning. We recognise that our students are a crucial workforce in leading and delivering person-centred practice.

The school's vision is to be world-leading in developing curricula to prepare healthcare professionals for person-centred practice. We have progressed a programme of learning, research and scholarly work that informs our approaches to facilitating learning in theory and practice. We are committed to leading this agenda to capitalise on the transformative impact of higher education in promoting the highest quality healthcare for patients, families, healthcare professionals and communities.

We believe that having shared values is fundamental to achieving our vision. Our team is invested in agreeing and reviewing our shared values as the basis for our ways of working. We strategically integrate the principles of person-centredness into healthcare curricula. Our work is underpinned by the Person-centred Nursing and Person-centred Practice Frameworks (McCance and McCormack 2021), which provide a conceptual overview of factors that collectively influence the achievement of person-centred outcomes and healthful cultures. Our local, national and international collaborations have enabled us to influence the development of person-centred healthcare professionals with the knowledge and skills to practise in person-centred ways. Our approach to operationalising person-centredness in healthcare curricula is illustrated in Figure 9.2.

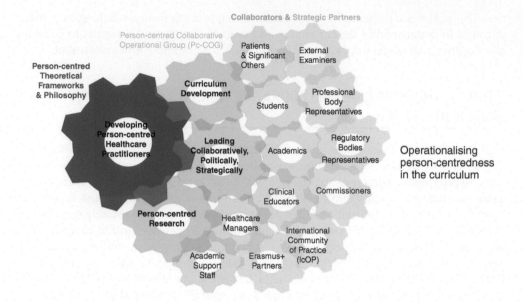

FIGURE 9.2   Partnership working with collaborators and strategic partners.

Through rich collaborative working, the team has led the design and delivery of a sustained programme of curriculum innovation. Acting as role models and change agents for person-centredness in healthcare curricula and practice has resulted in our School being ranked first in Ireland and seventh in the UK (www.ulster.ac.uk/faculties/life-and-health-sciences/nursing-paramedic-science). Working as a team, we have transformed the student learning experience by promoting the development of person-centredness in healthcare curricula. Our collaborative influence and impact are chronologically evidenced through:

- an award-winning, internationally significant doctoral participatory action research project that focused on how the caring attributes of undergraduate student nurses could be developed and sustained over time when students learnt in a programme grounded in person-centred principles (Cook et al. 2018). This resulted in the creation of the first regional, electronic, Northern Ireland Practice Assessment Document (e-NIPAD) based on the Person-centred Framework for Practice Learning and is now a regional learning and assessment tool
- leading, developing and implementing a novel person-centred app, which is used internationally to evidence nurses' unique contribution to patient and family experiences of care across healthcare settings (McCance et al. 2020)
- an award-winning, internationally important, doctoral mixed methods study demonstrating how, on completion of their studies, students' perceptions of their person-centred practice were improved, having experienced a PCC (O'Donnell 2021). The Person-centred Practice Inventory – Student Instrument developed and psychometrically tested as part of this research is the first theoretically derived instrument to measure students' perceptions of their person-centred

practice (O'Donnell et al. 2021). This instrument is being adapted for use in China, Norway, Sweden and Spain
■ receiving a UK Advance HE 2023 Collaborative Award for Teaching Excellence in recognition of our sustained, sector-leading work in promoting person-centredness in healthcare education, research and practice.

We utilise our influence, leadership and publications to drive a person-centred agenda, achieving fundamental changes in educational standards for healthcare education. Notably, the UK's Nursing and Midwifery Council standards explicitly emphasise the need for nurses to practise in person-centred ways (NMC 2018). Effecting change, our team modelled person-centred ways of being in renewing our undergraduate nursing curriculum, offering stakeholders exceptional support and fostering conditions for authentic collaboration. The curriculum renewal co-ordinator led the team to achieve NMC and University approval without conditions, an exceptional achievement accomplished by only four other universities nationally.

Through the work highlighted above, academic and practice learning experiences and outcomes have been enhanced. Our curricula reflect the application of person-centred principles to real-life healthcare practice with evidence of local, national and international impact. For example, learning experiences employ supportive, experiential and active learning pedagogies that prepare students for person-centred practice and future employability (Figure 9.3). This is endorsed by University metrics which show 100% employability of our nursing students. Additionally, postgraduate registered nursing students (2013–2020) undertaking our practice-based programmes have been promoted to senior leadership roles. In addition, in its quality standards audit, the

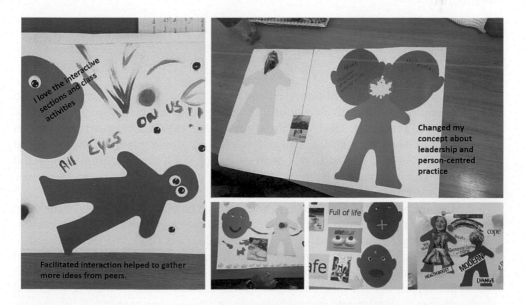

FIGURE 9.3   Using creativity to facilitate an understanding of person-centred practice.

Northern Ireland Practice Education Council highlighted our programme's 'quantifiable impact on service users'.

Having leading roles on regional workforce and education subgroups, team members have been instrumental in ensuring that person-centredness has shaped the Regional Nursing and Midwifery Strategy, as evidenced in strategic reports. This includes working with the Department of Health to lead the development of a Framework for Practice Learning into a digital platform for undergraduate student nurses (e-NIPAD portfolio educational tool). The project provided opportunities for team members, students, lecturers and practice partners to engage in focus groups to develop an electronic portfolio to support learning in both University and practice settings to demonstrate students' transformative learning against national standards. Since its launch in 2020, over 2500 undergraduate nursing students across Northern Ireland have used the portfolio to develop their proficiencies. The e-NIPAD is endorsed by the Department of Health and its 'valuable and innovative contribution to learning' has been commended by the NMC.

Drawing on our success, strong external networks and sustained commitment to developing pedagogical knowledge, we have shared our expertise transnationally by co-leading an international Erasmus+ project on person-centredness in healthcare curricula (2019–2023). Our collective leadership, mutuality and collaborative working enabled us to effectively work with five European partners (co-authors in this book) by engaging stakeholders through national and international consensus conferences in Ireland, the UK and Europe. With partners, we also co-led the development and delivery of two international development schools involving 68 participants from five countries to pilot and evaluate educational programmes to support educators to lead and facilitate person-centred curricula. Feedback from a participant highlighted:

> After going through the week's training and activities, I can say I am more confident in my practice as a person-centred learning facilitator. (Development school participant)

Finally, we have extended our reach and impact to enhance student learning and development by collaboratively publishing and editing six books underpinned by person-centred practice. Collectively, these books have 1539 citations and are key texts in multiple universities internationally. Developing a growing body of evidence and sharing initiatives are central to our progressive approach to curriculum design and delivery, to enhance student learning, drive policy change and impact on the future healthcare workforce.

Living out person-centred ideals is challenging. The team is conscious of the need to support new members of the education team to understand and work with person-centred philosophy and aligned pedagogic principles. We also recognise the need to remain committed to reflecting on how we are living out our person-centred ideals to create energy for innovation and to prevent us from becoming complacent.

Reflecting on our learning enables us to address challenges so that we work and learn together to develop and successfully deliver action plans to enhance the student learning experience. For example, our Competence Test Centre (CTC) is designed to assess international nurses' practice against the current UK pre-registration standards, requiring everyone to work with person-centred values to enable candidates to perform to the best of their ability. We worked closely with the CTC education team to agree principles of engagement (Chapter 5 Shared Values), to support a mutual understanding of person-centred ideals and empower them to create a supportive and person-centred learning environment. This included a review and redevelopment of the NMC Test of Competence which has led to a reduction in national appeals and complaints from over 400 per month to an average of one per month. This approach positively impacted the international student experience, further demonstrating how we role model person-centred behaviours in supporting learning and assessment.

> Staff have helped us to reduce our anxiety and provide us with the needed information. The assessor and the staff are so helpful, that helped me to face my worries. (CTC candidate)

By working collaboratively with our extensive partnership networks, and in leading pedagogic change, our collective excellence and reputation in person-centredness have been influential in transforming healthcare curricula. Developing a growing body of evidence and sharing initiatives are central to our progressive approach to embedding person-centredness in curriculum design and delivery. In so doing, we enhance student learning, drive policy change and develop the future healthcare workforce for person-centred practice.

For our team, person-centredness involves ways of being that value persons. This includes ensuring all voices are heard and consensus is reached through dialogue and shared decision making. Our authenticity in collaboration and our inclusive person-centred ways of working translate into healthful learning cultures and positive learning experiences.

> The whole teaching ethos is all around person-centredness. The course and all of the teaching is focused around person-centred care and we are constantly reminded of how you would do this in practice. The framework by McCormack and McCance just comes right into my head, straight away. The framework guides my thoughts. (Undergraduate nursing student)

The key message is that person-centredness in healthcare curricula has collaboration at its core. This aligns with our values and curricular philosophy that excellence is achieved through being together, working together and learning together.

In achieving our vision, we recognise the need to invest in people and partnerships to develop our ways of working and achieve meaningful impact. We remain committed to the further development of pedagogic research to support education for person-centred practice and to investigate the utility and impact of the PCCF on developing healthful learning cultures. As our team continues to evolve and expand, we recognise the need for leadership in prioritising the support and development of colleagues and partners (new and existing). We will continue to use collaborative approaches to channel our collective capacity in progressing person-centredness in healthcare curricula.

STORY 2: DEVELOPING A PERSON-CENTRED CULTURE IN EDUCATION – THE FACULTY OF HEALTH SCIENCES, UNIVERSITY OF MARIBOR STORY

Mateja Lorber, Gregor Štiglic, Sergej Kmetec.
In this story, Mateja, Sergej and Gregor reflect on how one faculty has worked to enable a person-centred culture to be developed. They reflect on their own personal journeys and those of a student (Ana).

MATEJA: Let's talk about the work we have been doing to develop our workplace culture in the Faculty. Gregor, I know you have reflected a lot on your own experience of becoming an educator and how that has evolved and developed for you. Can you share your story with us please?

GREGOR: Of course, and yes it has been an important experience to reflect on and share with you and others. During my time as an educator at a school of health sciences, I have experienced a transformative journey characterised by personal exploration, development and significant transformation. It all began with a simple yet powerful belief in the potential of shared values to shape curricula, influence lives and embrace the fundamental principles of person-centred education. As I stepped into the role of an educator for the first time, I was met with multiple eager and expectant faces. Amidst the excitement, I held close a vision driven by shared values that would serve as the guiding light for my teaching. These weren't just words; they embodied compassion, respect and empathy. My goal was clear: to make a place where the ties we made were more important than any rules and where each student's uniqueness was valued above all else.

MATEJA: I remember you sharing those values with me and also your passion for being an educator. How did you work with those values?

GREGOR: Well, it gradually dawned on me that our curriculum was not just a set of academic topics. Each passing day solidified the understanding that our curriculum was a complex weaving of shared values. My mission was to make these values palpable and infuse them into our programme's DNA. From the overarching philosophy to the smallest learning outcomes, the roots of our teachings were anchored firmly in the soil of person-centredness. I, along with my fellow educators, was not just an instructor; I had the privilege of nurturing personhood.

MATEJA: It is so true that our curriculum is more than a collection of topics, but making that real is a challenge for many educators. What was the key holding principle for you in achieving that?

GREGOR: Well, amidst this educational landscape, it struck me like lightning. The words of a fellow educator reverberated within me: 'Seeing someone holistically makes you see someone bigger too'. These words became a catalyst for a shift in perspective. Healthcare wasn't solely about treating ailments but forging connections, understanding narratives and looking beyond clinical symptoms. I understood that embracing this holistic outlook could mould students into healers capable of touching lives in ways beyond medical intervention.

MATEJA: That's a beautiful way of viewing education and healthcare, Gregor. How did you bring others along with you?

GREGOR: Navigating the journey wasn't without its challenges. Doubts often clouded my path, and the consistent alignment of values and actions felt daunting. However, these challenges ignited a fierce determination within me. I realised that actions spoke louder than words; I needed to demonstrate these values through my behaviour. Collaboratively, we began crafting manifestos that encapsulated the essence of person-centredness in our roles as educators, mentors and leaders. These documents became our compass, steering us through the uncharted waters of educational transformation.

MATEJA: What has been your key learning?

GREGOR: In retrospect, the evolution of my journey becomes evident. I've come to understand the power of embracing vulnerability and creating safe spaces for learners to explore the emotional dimension of education. Esteemed senior staff shared personal anecdotes, which became lessons in humility and resilience for our students. To my fellow educators, I extend a heartfelt call to action. Embrace shared values not merely as curriculum components but as the cornerstone of your purpose. Let them illuminate your interactions, guide your decisions and shape your pedagogy. The journey will be arduous, yet the lasting impact is immeasurable. Let's weave these values into our classrooms, creating a mosaic of positive change that touches students' lives, one by one. This is my journey – a narrative of discovering purpose in shared values.

I invite you to join me on this transformative path as we collectively shape the future through person-centred education.

GREGOR: Thanks for the opportunity to share my story, Mateja. It has been really helpful to reflect on these. But Mateja, you have been in the Faculty much longer than me and have been striving for this kind of culture with others too. You have reflected with Sergej on the way this culture has shaped learning with students. Can you share your reflections with us too?

SERGEJ: Yes, we reflected on many student experiences but one that stands out is that of Ana. Ana stepped into the dynamic world of healthcare education with us. Little did she know that this journey would shape her understanding of healthcare and redefine her perspective on leadership and learning. From the very beginning, Ana encountered a new world of systems. It wasn't just about textbooks and lectures but a sophisticated orchestration of teaching, learning, facilitation, assessment and evaluation methods. These systems were the gears that drove the engine of a PCC that viewed human beings not as mere students but as unique individuals with diverse stories and needs.

GREGOR: What happened?

MATEJA: Ana's first encounter with person-centred healthcare was like fresh air. It wasn't just about nursing knowledge but about fostering an environment where everyone could flourish. As she immersed herself in the curriculum, she witnessed how the leaders orchestrated a harmonious blend of co-operation and collaboration. The atmosphere was electric with a sense of purpose, as professors, practitioners and students collectively designed, delivered and evaluated educational programmes. It wasn't just a classroom, it was a shared mission.

SERGEJ: I remember that time so well! The concept of person-centredness became Ana's compass. It wasn't merely a philosophy but a way of approaching fellow human beings with care and empathy. Ana marvelled at how educators imparted nursing skills and honed the art of education. They guided students to think critically through insightful questions and reflective exercises, shaping them into well-rounded healthcare professionals.

MATEJA: Indeed. One key aspect that resonated deeply with Ana was the emphasis on being present and connected. The educators weren't just teaching; they were caring, empathetic leaders who embodied the values they taught. They listened intently, using their senses to understand the unique context of everyone's journey. Even when physically absent, their influence lingered, guiding students and stakeholders towards the shared vision. This genuine connection created a sense of belonging, motivating everyone to do their best. The concept of harmonising and aligning visions was an eye-opener for Ana. The leaders encouraged open dialogue in critical and creative spaces, nurturing an environment where shared values and beliefs took root. In these vibrant discussions, diverse perspectives collided and collaborated, igniting sparks of insight and innovation. Through action-oriented discourse, students like Ana learned that leadership wasn't about asserting authority but about inspiring unity through shared purpose.

GREGOR: But was it really that easy?

MATEJA: No, it wasn't easy at all. Ana discovered that true leadership involved balancing needs. The leaders constantly questioned conventional norms, seeking equilibrium between individual aspirations, collective goals and external regulations. The curriculum wasn't rigid; it evolved due to systematic evaluations that shed light on balancing priorities. Ana saw that true leaders navigated complexity with wisdom and adaptability. Perhaps the most profound lesson Ana learned was about reflexive leaders who, she observed, possessed the rare art of listening with their hearts. Their responsiveness wasn't just reactive, it was proactive. They adapted their positions to motivate continuous action, growth and development.

SERGEJ: I have an example of some of those challenges. One day, Ana found herself in a class that deviated from the plan. Rather than sticking to a rigid structure, the educators embraced adaptability and valued each student's individuality. Ana understood genuine education was about fostering connections and getting to know each student personally. This approach to teaching and learning encouraged vibrant discussions and nurtured a spirit of curiosity. The assessment took on a new meaning in this world. Ana encountered portfolio assessments that evaluated both formative and summative aspects. Rubrics were unambiguous, giving students a roadmap to success. The focus was on multiple assessment methods, catering to various learning styles and adapting to rapidly changing contexts.

GREGOR: Thanks for sharing that example as it shows how we need to embrace reflexivity to really engage in person-centred learning. Did Ana manage to embrace these ways of working for herself and in her unique way?

MATEJA and Sergej: Yes, she did, and it was wonderful to see that. Ana realised that person-centred healthcare wasn't just a curriculum – it was a way of life. Through the nurturing leadership of her mentors, she had not only imbibed medical knowledge but had also grown as a compassionate and insightful individual. She was now prepared to step into the healthcare world as a person-centred leader, ready to make a meaningful impact on patients' lives and the healthcare system.

Ana's story exemplifies the transformative power of person-centred leadership in healthcare education. It wasn't just about memorising facts but about creating an ecosystem where empathy, collaboration and growth thrived. Her journey was a testament to the fact that authentic leaders could inspire change, foster unity and better shape healthcare's future.

Gregor, Mateja and Sergej go on to reflect on the overarching messages arising from their collective stories.

MATEJA: Across each of our stories, there are common themes. Perhaps we could identify what these are. In doing that, it will enable us to plan for how we continue to develop our person-centred culture and not be complacent about it!

GREGOR: For me one key theme is the power of shared values. I have come to realise the profound impact that shared values can have on education. Values, like compassion, respect and empathy, are not just theoretical concepts but guiding principles that shape the entire educational experience. Our experiences show the potential for transformation when these values are integrated into the curriculum and teaching approach. Healthcare goes beyond treating physical symptoms and explicit shared values bring this to life in the curriculum. The shift in perspective towards holistic care, understanding narratives and forging connections underscores the transformational power of adopting a more comprehensive approach to education and healthcare.

SERGEJ: I would agree with that, and it links to a second theme that resonates with me – nurturing individuality. Our stories show the importance of cherishing each person's individuality, highlighting the importance of creating an environment where personal connections are prioritised over rules and every person's uniqueness is celebrated. Our stories serve as an inspiring illustration of how person-centred education transforms not only students' professional competencies but also all our personal growth and empathetic outlook. It highlights the potential of reflective practices, collaborative learning and adaptability. But of course, shared values are critical to individuality being considered as a part of a 'whole' where everyone can adapt by being supported in a safe environment.

MATEJA: That last point resonates with me, and I would suggest that another theme is that of creating safe spaces. The importance of creating safe spaces for emotional exploration is evident in all our stories. By sharing personal anecdotes and stories, we create an environment where educators and students can engage with the emotional dimensions of learning. This highlights the significance of empathy and emotional intelligence in education. Reflective practices and facilitated learning spaces are essential for all of our personal and professional growth. Encouraging students to explore their thoughts, emotions and experiences contributes to a deeper understanding of themselves and their future roles as healthcare professionals. But also, the power of collaborative learning, by engaging students in discussions and interactions with peers, educators and mentors, fosters a sense of community, encouraging the exchange of ideas and the development of well-rounded professionals. Educators are seen as facilitators and mentors rather than mere instructors. It highlights for me the importance of supporting educators' continuous development in person-centred teaching and learning methods for the success of a curriculum that is person centred.

GREGOR: That is such an important point, Mateja, and makes me think about culture and context in our organisations. Successfully implementing a PCC requires an institution-wide commitment. It involves educators, administrative support, practice educators and a comprehensive framework that aligns with the philosophy. Person-centred education should be adaptable to various cultural and contextual factors. In a culture that is committed to person-centred ways of working, potential obstacles, such as aligning values with actions, are seen as opportunities for growth and when embraced with determination, and in a safe context, challenges can lead to meaningful change and personal development.

MATEJA, Gregor and Sergej: Our final thoughts to everyone are that we want to emphasise the enduring impact of embracing shared values. While the journey may be challenging, the influence on students' and educators' lives is immeasurable. Positive change can be created through a philosophy of person-centred education. Educators need to make shared values the cornerstone of their purpose and work collectively to shape the future through person-centred education; essentially, embracing challenges, nurturing individuality and transforming education through holistic approaches are key.

STORY 3: BECOMING A PERSON-CENTRED LEADER – A PROGRAMME FOR HEALTHCARE LEADERS

Shaun Cardiff

Education programmes, whether they be delivered by a higher education institution or learning and development departments of healthcare organisations, are often of long standing but seldom static. They evolve in response to changing staff and learner profiles, organisational strategies, national policy, local stakeholder needs and healthcare and educational trends. This has also been true for the Bachelor of Management in Healthcare (BaMiH) curriculum at Fontys University of Applied Sciences in The Netherlands, whose learners are qualified health and social care practitioners wanting to become (better) formal leaders/managers.

In 2016 a planned renewal of the four-year BaMiH curriculum created an opportunity for the faculty to share and utilise their knowledge, ideas and products on person-centredness and person-centred practice. Person-centredness was already a core faculty value and starting to influence the organisational culture. While person-centred healthcare practice was being taught in the Bachelor of Nursing programme, the concept of person-centredness and person-centred leadership was new for the BaMiH team and curriculum. With the intention of exploring a more person-centred approach to educational practice and introducing person-centred leadership into the repertoire of leadership styles, transformations began primarily within the leadership programme and lecturer team.

The leadership programme transformation was quite radical as the team considered the meaning of person-centredness alongside adult and transformative learning theory. The focus of learner outcomes shifted from demonstrating application of existent theory to the development and demonstration of a (evolving) personal vision of 'good' leadership. These were presented in written form at the end of years 2 and 3 of the four-year bachelor curriculum, and the evolving clarity, scope and/or depth questioned in oral examinations. At the end of year 4, learners were expected to also illustrate how their personal vision influenced how they led their small research project and subsequent improvement plan. The opportunity for a personalised and transformational leadership journey was a frequently named claim in learner, mentor/preceptor and lecturer evaluations.

Assuming that we should relate to learners as persons of equal value, actively self-determining and/or (re-)negotiating their learning journey, the education team started their own developmental journey in considering how person-centredness should influence their educational practice. While learning outcomes were formulated to guide student learning and examination, it was decided that there should be no predetermined or fixed programme content or structure. Lecturers were faced with the challenge of no longer 'teaching' but rather themselves now 'leading' a group of leaners in a person-centred way, to facilitate their individual and group development. Each group regularly (re-)negotiated what and/or how they wanted to collectively learn. Consequently, collective leadership was no longer a narrative taught or read about, and the advantages and challenges became a lived experience.

This change to traditional education practice was positive in the sense of learning scope and freedom, but also created feelings of trepidation and fear. As learners became partners in the learning process, they missed being told what to learn and produce to pass formal examinations. Lecturers too had to review the fulfilment of their role when no lesson plans existed to tell them what and how to teach. To facilitate role development and embodying of person-centredness, the educator team were facilitated in critically and creatively exploring the leading of a learning group using the person-centred leadership framework (Figure 9.4) (Cardiff et al. 2018). Metaphorically speaking, they started to learn to choreograph a dance (the learning sessions and journey) while dancing with learners, reflexively responding to both individual and group performance. This contrasted with a traditional approach of choreographing the dance beforehand and instructing dancers as a group how to perform the dance.

As stated earlier, curricula are seldom static. In 2020 the BaMiH was faced with new challenges posed by forces within the macro- and meso-contexts. The healthcare context was changing, the national profile of healthcare leaders was changing and the university was implementing a 'flexible' approach to student education. Careful melding and blending of these influences with lessons learned from 2016 to 2020 resulted in a new leadership programme entitled 'Leading with Impact'. Learners were still expected to demonstrate a personal and evidence-informed vision for good leadership. However, they were now expected to demonstrate the ability to systematically and methodically study workplace culture, design a development plan, then lead and evaluate the execution of at least one action. They were also expected to study their own leadership development journey, presenting it systematically and methodically in narrative form, and use the findings to inform their future development plan.

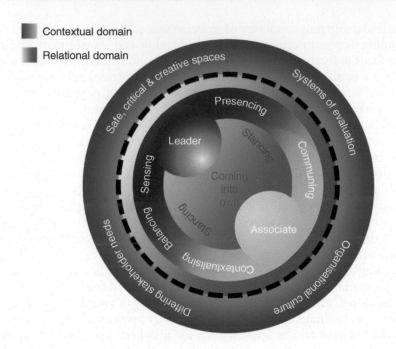

FIGURE 9.4   The person-centred leadership framework.
Source: Cardiff et al. (2018)/John Wiley & Sons.

The underlying philosophical and pedagogical principles for the leadership pro-gramme remained largely unchanged. However, a new challenge arose as learners were now also free to choose how they demonstrated learning outcomes, for instance, as written documents, a vlog, a face-to-face presentation or a portfolio assessment interview. Educators became concerned about how they could judge diverse products with equal rigour, and most learners felt over-challenged at having to decide how to demonstrate their learning outcomes. Pragmatism and co-constructivism lead to a con-sequent development of guidelines on how to demonstrate learning outcomes, which were welcomed and positively evaluated.

Another review with changes to the BaMiH curriculum can be expected in 2024. Stakeholder hopes, fears and expectations are already audible, and the leadership pro-gramme team have been gathering student feedback alongside their own observations and identification of current trends. For instance, systematically and methodically collecting data about their personal leadership development has proven to be a big challenge for most learners. Few collect data methodically and/or begin too late in the journey. A digital logbook/journal/planner is being developed with the criteria that it should offer sufficient structure to guide learner data gathering without hindering cre-ativity or flexibility and be incorporated into the existent digital learning environment.

The future is still bright, and our educational vision remains the same: enabling each learner to become the leader they need to be (for themselves, those they lead and the context in which they are leading) at this moment in their (working) life.

STORY 4: A NORWEGIAN PHD PROGRAMME IN PERSON-ORIENTED HEALTHCARE

Helle Kristine Falkenberg and Siri Tønnessen.
This story starts with the first PhD programme at the Faculty of Health and Social Sciences at the University of South-Eastern Norway (USN). The PhD programme focusing on person-oriented healthcare was the only one of its kind in Norway and was a key selling point in the Faculty study programme portfolio. After a merger of several departments, many academic staff and researchers felt that the focus of the programme did not suit them. The PhD programme was perceived as too nurse oriented, especially by many social scientists who struggled to find their place in the existing programme. It became apparent that a change was necessary.

The University board was clear that all faculties at the University should only have one PhD programme – and thus, it became necessary to develop a new PhD programme that would embrace everyone. A thorough process was initiated with a working group with participants from each department. They held meetings with all departments, research groups and research centres. The purpose was to find what united the various research areas at the faculty, to find a common platform from which to develop a new PhD. What was our unique selling point? After a longer person-centred process of involvement and feedback, the recognition of common ground between the person, health and society was identified.

At the same time, academic staff, students and leaders emphasised that many appreciated, and felt at home within, the person-centred perspectives. It was important strategically and emotionally that this was kept in the new PhD programme, and that we did not 'throw the baby out with the bathwater'. To ensure continuity in the transition, the initiative was taken to develop an elective course of five European study credits in person-oriented perspectives on research.

Two persons from the working group also participated at the same time in an Erasmus+ project on PCC development and saw the possibility of bringing more persons on board to develop a desirable person-centred course, for a broader audience. The Faculty therefore sent several academic staff from different disciplines to take part in activities organised by the E+ project, such as two international 5–7-day schools as well as the E+ digital course in person-oriented supervision. These staff were invited to participate in the development of the new PhD course, and to ensure that the course would be embraced broadly, to suit the Faculty's many different subjects and disciplines.

One major barrier to overcome was finding a common language that took into consideration different understandings related to language, terminology and concepts within different disciplines, to develop a shared understanding of how person-oriented perspectives embrace a wide range of research and education and, in its core value, is subject independent.

After a long process, we have succeeded in developing a course in person-oriented perspectives on research. To further strengthen the person-centred perspectives in the new PhD programme, the course has now been approved and made mandatory. This will promote a person-centred culture and continue this as the PhD programme's unique selling point.

Reflecting on our experience in the context of the PCC Framework, the story highlights many of the issues identified when we consider the curriculum 'structure'. But we believe that the experience of coming to a place of consensus exposed the relevance of the underpinning philosophical principles of the PCC Framework – transformative, relationalism, co-construction and pragmatism. The story happened because of the Faculty decision to terminate the PhD programme in person-oriented healthcare and establish a new programme that better captured and included new disciplines after a fusion of several departments at the Faculty of Health Sciences. The course aimed to ensure continuity of the person-centred perspectives already inherent in the existing programme. There was an overall understanding that person-centred perspectives should be continued, as they are relevant to many different healthcare professional groups and different areas of practice.

Various stakeholders in the old and new PhD programmes, including persons from the PhD programme board, course co-ordinators, PhD students, academic researchers, supervisors and educators, were involved in the process. All had experience and knowledge of person-centredness perspectives and the old PhD programme and this helped in reaching consensus. The stakeholders had several meetings and discussed how the person-centred perspectives could be made explicit and visible as a selling point in the new PhD programme. After close consideration and discussions, it became clear that the best option was to offer a 5 ECTS course in person-centred perspectives in research.

The stakeholders came together to develop the course and participated in the Erasmus+ project (PCC development) as project partners. One important strategic measure was to participate with several different staff in the Erasmus+ activities such as the two facilitators' and curriculum leaders' development schools. Another measure was to send learners to the development of a 5 ECTS digital course on person-centred doctoral supervision together with the other national Erasmus+ partners. The stakeholders developed a course curriculum according to the USN PhD course regulations, with relevant person-centred learning outcomes and student activities.

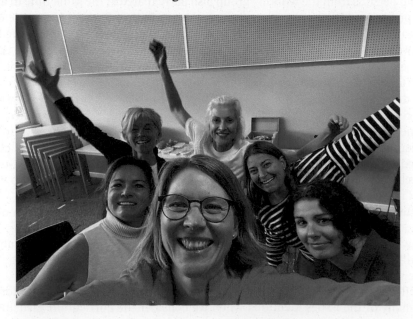

The new course has been accredited by the University as a 5 ECTS mandatory course in the new PhD programme. Participants from the various activities have contributed to the development of the course, and several have agreed to continue the work by taking part as facilitators and co-ordinators of the new course. Another success is that the person-centred perspectives are explicitly stated in the description of the new PhD in person, health and society study programme. Challenges have been related to language and culture relating to person-centred terminology, and that some understand person-centredness as mainly relevant to the nursing profession and science. This has been considered a major limitation to broadening its scope and acceptance by some departments in the Faculty of Health and Social Sciences. This was the main reason for the decision to develop a new PhD programme. Further attention needs to be given to promoting a person-centred culture, and to making visible how the 7S framework and values are currently embodied and can be understood in our curriculum.

Key learning from this work is that person-centred perspectives are still relevant and valued in the curriculum and are a unique selling point of the PhD programme. However, it is complex, and requires continuous development to broaden its understanding among the different stakeholders. The process required time to involve all stakeholders and their perspectives, to come to shared values and enable a course that is truly co-constructed in structure and substance. It is fundamental that the person-centred perspective is embedded in the leadership culture, to facilitate success. Further, it is important to involve people with different professional backgrounds.

STORY 5: LECTURERS AND LEADERS AS AMBASSADORS OF PERSON-CENTREDNESS IN THE FACULTY

Famke van Lieshout.
In 2022, having completed the international schools developed under the Erasmus+ project, a group of lecturers and team leaders agreed to join as ambassadors, to enable support and facilitation of person-centred curricula in the Faculty of People and Healthcare Studies at Fontys University of Applied Sciences, The Netherlands.

With person-centred practice already embedded in the Bachelor of Nursing (BaN) programme and an active knowledge centre for person-centred practices, the concept of person-centredness was not entirely new for the ambassadors. However, person-centredness was mainly connected with person-centred care relationships in education programmes. Consequently, students or faculty members rarely contemplated or discussed the meaning of person-centredness for other relationships such as learning relationships and working relationships, as well as the processes and structures associated with education and teamwork.

Motivations and drivers for the ambassadors are presented in Table 9.2.

Enabling the embodiment and embeddedness of person-centredness would not only increase credibility of the organisation's ambition to educate person-centred professionals, but also enable learners and staff to experience and live this value in their relationships, thereby fostering healthful workplace and learning cultures. In the spirit of building collective leadership, the 10 ambassadors approached the recently

TABLE 9.2 Motivations and Drivers for Developing the Ambassador Role.

- Person-centredness had been a Faculty core value for quite some time, but rarely discussed in terms of how it was influencing the realisation of the Faculty strategic vision.
- A fast-approaching review of the Bachelor in Nursing programme in response to a renewed National Nursing Education Profile.
- A restructuring of education staff whose home base was the BaN, resulting in the formation of six new teams, each with their own cohorts of students, clinical placement settings and area of expertise.
- Some individual ambassadors were already tasked with creating person-centred learning and work environments, by the Faculty's Board of Directors.

appointed 'craftsmanship' team who were tasked with advising teams and management on how to enact and embed the Faculty strategic plan.

As living one's core values is important to developing effective workplace cultures, the ambassadors started their development journey by reflecting on the meaning of person-centredness for their own practice. Everyday teaching and teamwork became the practice settings for testing assumptions and observing effects. They took advantage of all opportunities by taking a (leadership) position to present their work or perspectives and to invite people to look at what they were doing/wanted to do, through a person-centred lens. They consistently named and sometimes discussed person-centredness during formal and informal meetings. This not only aided the ambassadors in making person-centredness more tangible and unambiguous, but it also helped make it transparent and explicit for learners and other stakeholders. Often, actions could be agreed upon which would contribute to the development of person-centred learning and workplace environments.

Gradually, educators, (student) coaches, leaders and managers became increasingly aware of the significance of person-centredness for their relationships with each other, learners and colleagues connected to the design, delivery and evaluation of the curriculum.

The ambassadors' development felt daunting as they were to explore their own person-centredness while fostering it in others and within various environments. This required thorough understanding of person-centredness, sensitivity to identifying opportunities for person-centredness, leadership and facilitation. Two experts in person-centred practice were coupled with the group ambassadors to act as critical companions, facilitating understanding and embodiment through (strategic) meetings and coaching on the job. Meetings were held every four weeks and active learning methods were used to work through issues or questions and referenced to the PCC Framework.

A realisation started to emerge that various trends in higher education and healthcare practice were starting to show (un)intended fits with one or more of the 7S descriptors in the PCC framework. Referring to these trends and working with their initiatives could also become a vehicle for demonstrating the relevance of person-centredness. However, timely, insightful and carefully phrased contributions were needed if person-centredness was to be linked to these trends as they rarely focused beyond the design of an educational intervention or tool.

To prevent person-centredness becoming overshadowed by a pragmatic drive for interventions and tools, the ambassadors used a specific programme design to agree on a shared focus and to pool and structure their joint activities. This design was also used to capture the descriptors and tools they were using or had developed, and create action plans on what to do next. It also helped them visualise what they were doing, making it more tangible for management and other collaborators.

To widen their source of support and inspiration, the ambassador group encouraged one member to represent them within a person-centred practice global network (PCP-ICOP; www.pcp-icop.org), and they approached other international university teams who may be interested in forming a learning community on working with the PCC framework. The team of ambassadors now have a set of actions they are taking forward collaboratively, including:

- inviting teams to critically develop or review their own vision and strategy
- promoting and facilitating the development of person-centred leadership among those holding strategic positions within the Faculty, educational programmes and practice organisations associated with the curricula, helping them develop person-centred workplace and learning cultures
- using a practice development/participatory action research approach to developing person-centred curricula
- using the PCC Framework to screen and evaluate curricula
- collecting best practices for person-centred learning, collaboratively reflecting on why they are person centred and successful. This would then enable a more contextualised use within Faculty curricula
- remaining connected with small initiatives in programmes and pooling the findings using a programmatic approach.

STORY 6: A SLICE OF CAKE TO DEVELOP SAFE SPACES FOR LEARNING AND DEVELOPMENT

Caroline A.W. Dickson.

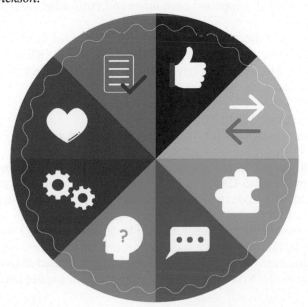

The PCC Framework emphasises the fundamental need to create person-centred learning environments if learners – students and educators – are to flourish. The focus of this story is on how a digital resource, CAKE, has been implemented to develop university and clinical educator colleagues in clinical supervision and in university and clinical workplaces.

My colleague Kath MacDonald, honorary lecturer at Queen Margaret University, and I embarked on a journey which began in 2020 to work collaboratively with healthcare students and professionals to develop a resource to support well-being. Initially, the intention was to promote well-being in clinical practice, but subsequently it has been used in university settings. Drawing on our expertise in storytelling and practice development, in phase 1 of the project we co-designed the prototype resource with eight nurses working in community settings. The initial prototype CAKE (**C**reating connections, **A**ttending to what's important, **K**eeping Connected, **E**nabling and empowering) had seven slices. The slices would lead teams through a process of creating a safe space for sharing stories of practice; storytelling using creative means such as modelling, drawing, painting, reflecting in nature; reflecting and action planning and evaluation (Dickson and MacDonald 2023).

There were three aims in phase 2 of the project. First, drawing on Hardiman and Dewing's (2014) critical ally model of facilitation, we developed 17 clinical leaders to become facilitators of CAKE. Facilitators were prepared and supported to implement CAKE with 130 health and social care practitioners, and we used multiple, creative methods of data collection to test the initial feasibility of CAKE. In 2022 a digital version of CAKE was created to be freely available to teams (www.listenupstorytelling.co.uk/welcome-to-cake/). The final version of CAKE has eight slices: Checking In; Checking Out; Shared Ways of Working; Creating a Shared Purpose, Storytelling; Reflection; Action Planning; and Evaluation.

The evaluation reinforced the need to create safe spaces for colleagues to share stories, but in the sharing of stories, teams began to know each other better as people, became more connected, supported each other and embedded well-being practices in their everyday work.

Since the initial evaluation, we have introduced CAKE to colleagues, educators in universities and practice and learners. We aimed to use CAKE with colleagues as a strategy to develop a healthy work environment. The two distinct aims of introducing CAKE to learners were to:

- develop their leadership of culture change
- use CAKE as a framework for clinical supervision in practice.

Two cohorts of community nursing learners undertaking a professional postgraduate degree were introduced to CAKE in an interactive workshop. The aim of the workshop was twofold: to introduce CAKE and help them familiarise themselves with the resource, and to develop their skills of person-centred facilitation. We gave an overview of the resource and some background on its development. We went through each slice, modelling facilitation. As we progressed through the slices, we invited learners to co-facilitate and then facilitate. After each slice, we discussed shared learning of the process, giving attention to facilitation tools, strategies and ways of being. We ended the workshop by considering how they would embed CAKE in the teams they led. CAKE is now being embedded across teams in partner organisations.

The story of CAKE focuses on how the resource can develop facilitation skills. It highlights the importance of creating a safe learning environment and paying attention to experiential learning – emotionality impacting on cognitive development. It also encourages learners to develop skills in reflexivity to be better able to deal with and address challenges in clinical practice.

STORY 7: ASSIGNMENT WRITING AS TRANSFORMATIVE LEARNING

Erna Haraldsdottir.
This story relates to implementing a person-centred written assignment into the curriculum of a core unit of learning (Theory and Practice of Person-centredness) in a Master's programme in person-centred practice. The Master's programme is a cross-disciplinary programme in the School of Health Sciences at Queen Margaret University and includes nursing, occupational therapy, art therapies and mad studies. This story illustrates how the structure of an assignment creates conditions for transformative learning and practice (Chapter 3 – Structure, in the 7S Framework). The assignment is an example of how an education team challenged the traditional system (Chapter 4 – System, in the 7S Framework) and created a flexible approach to the assignment with overarching guidelines and structure to foster meaningful and transformative learning.

The assignment is focused on the students demonstrating enhanced understanding of person-centred theoretical knowledge that can be applied to their own practice and is context specific to each student. The first part of the assignment invites the students to map current practice with person-centred theory or aspects of a person-centred theory. This is a creative and intellectual process of engaging with the learning and teaching content of the module and critical reflection of one's own practice. The students use a portfolio of learning to hold the material generated in this process to evidence their discovery.

> The structure of the assignment directs the students towards transformative learning through critical exploration of key materials in the context of their own practice.

The second part of the assignment is informed by the first part whereby the student, based on the discovery within the mapping processes, chooses a focus of the assignment that is relevant for their context and will support ongoing transformation of themselves as practitioners and their practice. The students are supported through the unit of learning with targeted content. The structure of the assignment directs the students towards transformative learning through critical exploration of key materials in the context of their own practice. The assignment is designed in such a way that there is no 'short cut' to writing without embodying the knowledge of the unit of learning content and applying it to contextual knowledge and understanding of self and own practice.

This is not without challenges for the students. The structure of the assignment requires them to be intellectually curious and creative and engage actively with the practical application of person-centred theory. Furthermore, they are encouraged to trust the process of discovery that will lead to successful assignment outcomes. Many students find this challenging in the beginning and struggle with the flexible nature of the assignment structure without a prescribed approach guiding the overall focus of the assignment. Some students get fixed around choosing the topic too early to reduce and manage 'assignment anxiety' which inhibits their thinking and being true to the process of discovery in mapping their own practice context. For the module team, there has been a need to support students and facilitate the process, but once the student understands and engages with the flexibility and the creative and analytical nature of the assignment, they are excited by the practice and practical applications of their learning.

It is very evident that students need to let go of old habits of traditional essay writing and to engage with the learning unit content. With support from the teaching and learning team, most students successfully achieve an increased understanding and the emergence of new insights that shape their assignment focus and writing style.

REFLECTING ON THESE MOTIVATIONAL STORIES

The worldwide vision to humanise healthcare and reorientate it to become more person centred calls for education that supports healthcare professionals to be reflexive, working within and influencing healthcare systems beyond the traditional boundaries (Phelan et al. 2020). Consequently, there is a need to reorientate the workforce, creating and enabling environments for transformational change and developing leaders and managers to support this (WHO 2007). The PCC Framework is a theoretical template that can be applied in practice to support and inform the education of healthcare professionals who can take an active part in influencing and leading the transformation of healthcare.

Although the work underpinning these stories was undertaken prior to the development of the PCC Framework, all of them provide details about how we can make sense of the PCC Framework as a whole and bring to life its different components.

The stories provide specific examples of how departments in different cultures and contexts adopt person-centred approaches in their various development activities. While the individual components of the stories in themselves may not be radical or unusual, it is the connections and challenges made through these connections that enable person-centred perspectives to emerge. Addressing the development needs of staff is a significant focus of several stories. These stories illustrate how within the university context, the development of PCC starts with the transformation of the programme team who are developing the curriculum. While there is a commitment to person-centredness in many universities, the understanding of what it means in a curriculum context is not always realised in practice. We see examples of the processes of transformation for curriculum teams as they explore the meaning of person-centredness in relation to leading teaching and learning.

It is often the case that we try to develop innovations by employing the same methods we always have and then wonder why they didn't work or were not sustained! Leadership is one of those practices that often needs a radical alteration for new practices in and among teams to surface. Teams need to engage with a fresh perspective on leadership to underpin teaching and engage with new theories in relation to person-centred leadership. In these stories, we see new approaches to exploring person-centred leadership, shifting the focus of outcome from fixed knowledge generation to an evolving vision of 'good' leadership informed by person-centredness. The transformation in story 3, for example, reflects one of the core principles of person-centred curricula, that students are not told what to learn but are invited to engage with the learning and teaching programme. We also see this evidenced in Story 2. This engagement challenges traditional hierarchies of lecturer (as expert) and student (as passive) and instead places learners in a position of equal value, actively self-determining and/or (re-)negotiating their learning journey. The learning is transformative, lived through experience and contextualised to each individual learner.

We also see stories of challenging dominant pedagogical approaches, especially relating to how we determine if learning has taken place. Too often in education assessment, essay writing is a dominant activity, with an expectation that learners can join up the focus of different essays and other assignments and apply it to their ongoing learning and development. We know that this is a challenge for many learners, and so using approaches to assessment that 'scaffold' the development of their knowledge and build it into a portfolio of evidence actively facilitates analysis and synthesis of learning that can be more easily applied in practice. We see further evidence in these stories of the adoption of creative and innovative approaches to engagement, facilitation and assessment of learning. Doing this can be challenging as the knowledge, skills and expertise of academic staff may not have been developed beyond the more standardised methods. Therefore, if we are going to challenge assessment methods and develop more alternative approaches, staff development is critical.

> Key message 1: In shifting the curriculum from more traditional approaches to those that are more person centred, starting with the transformation of the curriculum team may be a key step and this is consistent with the 'Style' and 'Skills' components of the Person-centred Curriculum Framework.

It is not unusual for universities as complex systems to engage in reorganisation of structures and systems to keep abreast of societal change. So, while a curriculum development may have served a particular purpose, organisational change may challenge this purpose and curriculum change becomes necessary. Such reorganisations not only challenge curriculum structures and processes but also the whole basis of the curriculum and its relevance to different stakeholders. Consistent with what we know from the literature, definitions and meanings of person-centredness differ and finding common ground is a challenge. While this challenge of reaching consensus about the meaning of person-centredness, person-centred healthcare and person-centred practice is recognised in the literature, story 4 shows how the same lack of consensus can permeate the curriculum.

Developing shared values has been shown in several stories to be a critical 'anchor' in enabling respectful, inclusive and innovative conversations. It is important for a curriculum development team to find common ground and a shared vision that will underpin curriculum development. This is especially the case when a programme is shared between many faculties across an institution. In the stories told in this chapter, we see examples of finding this common ground through specific units of study as a shared place for engagement, through staff reflexivity resulting in their own learning and transformation, finding common language and creating shared understandings of concepts and terminology used. Demonstrating the importance of the work of the curriculum team to develop these foundations seems to be a good first step in the curriculum development process.

Key message 2: Taking the time to develop shared values as a starting point in curriculum change or innovation is key. These shared values act as an anchor for all ongoing changes, developments and innovations and link directly with the 'shared values' component of the PCC Framework.

Flexibility and trust in the process of teaching and learning are core concepts in person-centred curricula. 'Holding' learners through what may appear to them as unstructured and non-prescribed teaching, learning and assessment processes is challenging. While adult education methodologies are advocated and encouraged in most professional development programmes, students often find these 'novel' methods to be anxiety provoking.

A critical issue for all of us to consider is how we determine if learning has occurred and how we assess that. As noted earlier, traditional essay writing is often overused as an assessment method and in several of the stories in this chapter, we see how other methods support and encourage transformation of learners and their practice. Instead of the assessment being a predetermined outcome-oriented approach, we see learners being encouraged and enabled to contextualise and embed their learning in choosing both the assessment focus and its method of completion. Many students find this challenging, especially those who are used to the more traditional essay writing. The key to success in adopting more creative and self-directed assessment methods is for learners to be supported to trust the process that is less prescribed, more fluid in its operation and negotiated with others. Doing this helps learners to engage with learning methodologies that are co-created and have the transformative intent of challenging taken-for-granted assumptions and their potential to create change in their work context that is more person centred.

We can never overemphasise the importance of doing the groundwork needed for PCC development. Key to this is generating shared understanding of person-centredness. As with many organisations, there is always some understanding of person-centredness that may drive curriculum development but there is a need for ongoing engagement in order for person-centredness to be truly embedded in curricula. The sustained development demonstrated in Story 1 clearly shows the need for organisational commitment to culture change. The collective actions of a team of people with a shared vision and values are clearly evidenced and materialised into a sophisticated PCC. It is a powerful story of how a curriculum reflecting all the 7Ss of the PCC

Framework can be operationalised in practice. Their story shows how eventually all the efforts and approaches described within the other stories in this chapter come together and how micro-level actions can influence a PCC being designed as a whole system and delivered at a macro-level.

> Key message 3: Creating a person-centred whole-systems approach to curriculum development is not a linear or one-off process or event. Micro-level small-scale steps to a more person-centred approach can be scaled through systematic approaches to learning and development that are embedded in facilitative processes of engagement.

Reflecting on these stories, the focus on continuous system and team developments has been emphasised. While it is easy to espouse person-centred principles, values and philosophies in a written curriculum document that can lead to accreditation, it is another thing entirely to translate those principles, values and philosophies into embodied and embedded practices. Formal development processes and programmes may be necessary to act as catalysts for change and innovation. These learning opportunities (in the form of formal programmes of study) provide safe spaces for brave conversations, where everyone taking part can be helped to look deeply at the realities of (their) practice. As facilitators of PCC implementation, then, we need to engage with both our own transformation and that of others we engage and work with, so as to make person-centredness real in the curriculum.

Such programmes can take many forms and several stories in this chapter highlight different approaches taken to achieving a transformational outcome. As reflected in these stories, the core condition for a PCC starts with the team which develops the curriculum. Formal processes of transformative learning provide structures and systems that create the conditions for participants to connect emotionally, engage in critical and creative transformative processes, and experience embodied ways of being and doing that become the basis for ongoing innovative approaches to teaching, learning and assessment in the curriculum. But participating in such programmes is not enough and it is the ongoing reflexive commitment to the transformation of self and others that eventually results in a change of perspective and a shift towards a PCC as a whole system.

> Key message 4: When embarking on the journey of developing a PCC, it is important to consider the available knowledge, skills and expertise of team members and the need for formal development. Such formal development has the potential to shift perspectives for individuals, teams and organisations.

Such commitment has a ripple effect, as the conscious living out of values of compassion, respect and empathy can influence individuals who together can develop a collective manifesto for organisational change. Several stories that have this kind of focus highlight the importance of embracing vulnerability, doubts and emotions and being resilient in the quest towards truly living our values. However, these stories also are committed to transferring that development into action with learners and achieving person-centred learning outcomes.

SUMMARY

In this chapter we have presented seven stories that show the different approaches that can be adopted towards the development and implementation of a PCC. As stated at the outset, these stories are not meant to be 'ideals' nor exhaustive in demonstrating the potential for PCC development. However, they do demonstrate the courage and commitment of those who have undertaken this work. When engaging in such developments, we know that there are many obstacles and challenges, and we also know that it can feel like a very lonely experience. The development and implementation of a PCC is essentially an exercise in culture change, and we know that it is not a one-off project or course. Instead, it requires an ongoing commitment from curriculum leaders to be critical and creative, to show vulnerability, to embrace difference and to be willing to let go of the many 'sacred cows' we all hold in our individual mental models of 'what is best'. Nobody embarks on this kind of work if they are not passionate about person-centred cultures and committed to those ways of knowing, being and doing for the transformation of self and others – especially future person-centred healthcare practitioners.

    The four key messages derived from these stories can be seen as building blocks for embarking on this journey and we bring these together in Figure 9.5 and offer them as a framework for reflection and planning that may help the journey of transformation begin.

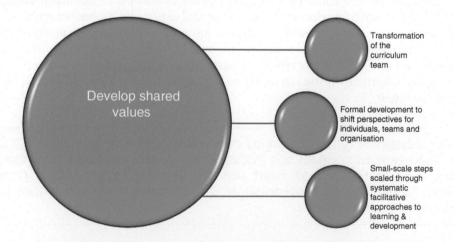

FIGURE 9.5   Framework for reflecting and planning person-centred curriculum implementation.

REFERENCES

Cardiff, S., McCormack, B., and McCance, T.V. (2018). Person-centred leadership: a relational approach to leadership derived through action research. *Journal of Clinical Nursing* 27: 3056–3069.

Cook, N.F., McCance, T., McCormack, B. et al. (2018). Perceived caring attributes and priorities of pre-registration nursing students throughout a nursing curriculum underpinned by person-centredness. *Journal of Clinical Nursing* 27 (13–14): 2847–2858.

Dickson, C.A.W. and MacDonald, K. (2023). Embedding storytelling in practice through CAKE – a recipe for team well-being and effectiveness. *International Practice Development Journal* 13 (1): 3.

Hardiman, M. and Dewing, J. (2014). Critical ally and critical friends: stepping stones to facilitating practice development. *International Journal of Practice Development* 4 (1): 1–19.

McCance, T. and McCormack, B. (2021). The person-centred nursing framework. In: *Person-Centred Nursing Research: Methodology, Methods and Outcomes* (ed. J. Dewing, B. McCormack, and T. McCance), 13–28. Switzerland: Springer.

McCance, T., Lynch, B., Boomer, C. et al. (2020). Implementing and measuring person-centredness using an APP for knowledge transfer: the iMPAKT app. *International Journal of Quality in Healthcare* 32 (4): 251–258.

Nursing and Midwifery Council (2018). *Future Nurse: Standards of Proficiency for Registered Nurses*. London: Nursing and Midwifery Council.

O'Donnell, D. (2021). Becoming a Person-centred Healthcare Professional: A Mixed Methods Study. Doctoral thesis, Ulster University.

O'Donnell, D., Slater, P., McCance, T. et al. (2021). The development and validation of the person-centred practice inventory – student instrument: a modified Delphi study. *Nurse Education Today* 100: 104826.

Phelan, A., McCormack, B., Dewing, J. et al. (2020). Review of developments in person-centred healthcare. *International Practice Development Journal* 10, article 3.

World Health Organization (2007). People-centred Healthcare: A Policy Framework. www.who.int/publications/i/item/9789290613176

RESOURCES

CAKE Facilitation Workshops: www.listenupstorytelling.co.uk/cake-facilitation-workshops/

Index

A

action-oriented staff meeting, 187
active learning, 203–204
appreciative inquiry (AI), 202

B

Bachelor of Management in Healthcare
    (BaMiH) curriculum, 234
Bachelor of Nursing (BaN), 239

C

claims, concerns and issues (CCI), 204–205
coaching, 175–176
co-constructed curriculum, 64–65
Collaborative Award for Teaching Excellence
    (CATE), 227
Competence Test Centre (CTC), 228, 229
courageous conversations, 119
    attentive, 120
    demonstrating integrity, 119
    intentions, 118
craftsmanship, 240
Creating connections, Attending to what's
    important, Keeping Connected,
    Enabling and empowering
    (CAKE), 241–243
critical companionship model, 206
critical reflexive collaborative learning, 182
critical reflexive learning, 23
curriculum framework
    principles, 5–8
    7s framework methodologies
        shared values, 21–22
        skills, 22–23
        staff, 23
        strategy, 17–19

        structure, 19–20
        style, 22
        systems, 20–21

E

educators, 19, 21, 22, 87, 94, 96, 130
embedding shared values, 123–125
    recruitment and selection, 125
    in staff appraisals, 127
    in staff induction, 126–127
    in whole-system approach, 125–127
e-NIPAD portfolio educational tool, 228
Erasmus programmes, 82

F

facilitation, 194
    person-centred, 165, 242
    skills
        active learning, 203–204
        appropriate facilitation strategy, 198
        critical companionship model, 206
        delivery of, person-centred
            education, 207–208
        exploring curriculum, 201
        participation, 198–200
        playfulness and creative approaches, 205
        reflexivity and reflection, 203
facilitator(s), 161
feedback
    action planning tool, 180
    criticism, 122–123
    giving and receiving, 120, 124
    successful feedback, 123
flourish-o-meter, 185–186
Fontys University of Applied Sciences, 239–241
full-time equivalent (FTE), 172